O A P L
OXFORD AMERICAN PAIN LIBRARY

Back and Neck Pain

Bill H. McCarberg, MD
Practitioner, Family Medicine
Founder, Chronic Pain Management Program
Kaiser Permanente
San Diego, California

Steven Stanos, DO
Medical Director
Center for Pain Management
Rehabilitation Institute of Chicago
Chicago, Illinois

Yvonne D'Arcy, MS, CRNP, CNS
Pain Management and Palliative Care Nurse Practitioner
Suburban Hospital
Johns Hopkins Medicine
Bethesda, Maryland

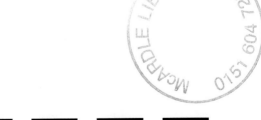

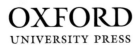

OXFORD
UNIVERSITY PRESS

OXFORD
UNIVERSITY PRESS

Oxford University Press, Inc., publishes works that further
Oxford University's objective of excellence
in research, scholarship, and education.

Oxford New York
Auckland Cape Town Dar es Salaam Hong Kong Karachi
Kuala Lumpur Madrid Melbourne Mexico City Nairobi
New Delhi Shanghai Taipei Toronto

With offices in
Argentina Austria Brazil Chile Czech Republic France Greece
Guatemala Hungary Italy Japan Poland Portugal Singapore
South Korea Switzerland Thailand Turkey Ukraine Vietnam

Copyright © 2012 by Oxford University Press, Inc.

Published by Oxford University Press, Inc.
198 Madison Avenue, New York, New York 10016
www.oup.com

Oxford is a registered trademark of Oxford University Press

Library of Congress Cataloging-in-Publication Data

McCarberg, Bill H.
Back and neck pain / Bill H. McCarberg, Steven Stanos, Yvonne D'Arcy.
p. ; cm. — (Oxford American pain library)
Includes bibliographical references and index.
ISBN 978-0-19-539457-3 (pbk. : alk. paper)
I. Stanos, Steven. II. D'Arcy, Yvonne M. III. Title. IV. Series: Oxford American
pain library.
[DNLM: 1. Back Pain—diagnosis—Handbooks. 2. Back Pain—therapy—Handbooks.
3. Neck Pain—diagnosis—Handbooks. 4. Neck Pain—therapy—Handbooks. WE 39]
LC-classification not assigned
617.5'6406—dc23   2011028818

9 8 7 6 5 4 3 2 1
Printed in the United States of America
on acid-free paper

Disclosures

Dr. McCarberg has received honorarium from Pricara, Forest, and NeurogesX.

Dr. Stanos has consulted and has been a speaker for Endo Pharmaceuticals, King Pharmaceutical, Lilly, Forest, Ortho-McNeil/Pricara, Pfizer, and Purdue. He was also a consultant for MyMatrix and Wellpoint

Ms. D'Arcy has consulted for Ortho-McNeil/Pricara, Archimedes, Zogenix, and Pfizer, and she currently serves on the Pfizer speakers' bureau.

Preface

Low back pain is such a common occurrence that most Americans experience it at some time in their adult lives. In a study with 31,044 patients, about one-fourth of the adult American population reported experiencing low back pain in the 3 months prior to the study.[1] Between the two types of pain, neck and back, Americans experience pain disability and decreased quality of life in record numbers, and many try to self-treat before seeking help from their health care provider.

Because these two types of pain have such a negative impact on patients with high resource utilization costs, it is important for health care providers to understand the causes and treatment options for these conditions. There is no aspect of the patient's life that is unaffected when a patient has back or neck pain, so a comprehensive treatment plan is needed. At least one in eight patients with low back pain loses time away from work, and presenteeism is a growing problem. Working while in pain can affect not only job performance but the ability of the patient to retain his or her job.

It is my hope that this book will help health care providers who care for these patients better understand the two conditions and utilize the research base that provides direction for treatment options. Managing back and neck pain not only requires medication management but also the use of behavioral, complementary, and other types of integrative techniques can be helpful adjuncts to medications. It is my hope that this book will encourage health care providers of all types to use the information in this book to help these patients with their very difficult-to-manage pain.

Yvonne D'Arcy, MS, CRNP, CNS

References

1. Barnes P, Powell-Griner E, McFann K, Nahin R. Complementary and Alternative Medicine Use among Adults: United States, 2002. NCCAM, May 2004.

Contents

Contributor

Anjum Sayyad, MD
PM&R Resident
Rehabilitation Institute of Chicago
Chicago, IL

Chapter 1

Introduction

Bill McCarberg

Back and neck pain are common and affect 60% to 80% of the population at some time during their lives,[1] with acute back pain affecting up to 44% of the working population each year.[2] In the United States, back and neck pain (both acute and chronic) are the second most common neurological complaints after headache.[3] The National Health and Nutrition Education Survey (NHANES) showed that over a 6-month period, 59 million people in the United States had acute or chronic back pain.[4]

Back and neck pain are also very common in the primary care setting. It has been reported to be the sixth most common reason for physician visits among patients 17–44 years of age, fifth for patients 45–64 years old, and eighth in patients ≥65 years of age.[5] The prevalence rates are as high as 40% in Western Europe, with men and women affected equally.[6] Prevalence also increases with age and is highest among those 70 to 79 years old.[2] Factors, in addition to advancing age, that are associated with increased risk for back and neck pain include poor physical fitness; smoking; obesity; weakness of back, neck, and abdominal muscles; and occupational factors (e.g., heavy work, lifting, bending, pulling).[7]

The costs associated with this condition are substantial. In 2004, the estimated annual direct cost of treating back pain in the United States was $193.9 billion ($638 per person in the population). In addition, annual indirect costs for lost wages resulting from back pain were $22.4 billion.[7] Results from the United States National Ambulatory Medical Care Survey showed 61.7 million office visits for acute and chronic back pain in 2003; of these, 42.4 million were in primary care.[8] The average number of lost workdays per occurrence was 7.2 among 25.9 million workers for a total of 186.7 million days in 2003.[9]

Absenteeism is a well-known consequence of neck and back pain. Presenteeism is a newer concept. At a major U.S. corporation, the most common health conditions causing at-work impairment were allergies, joint pain, and back or neck disorders. Decreases in on-the-job work functioning due to these conditions ranged from 17.8% to 36.4%, and the overall costs linked to presenteeism exceeded those of absenteeism and medical treatment combined.[10] Kaiser Permanente found that back pain was the fourth-leading cause of presenteeism productivity losses after depression, fatigue, and sleeping problems.[11]

Acute back and neck pain are usually self-limited, with symptomatic treatment resulting in resolution. Despite a growing knowledge about pathophysiology, persistent pain management is difficult. Primary care providers struggle with unexplained variability among pain patients. Physical abnormalities are not predictive of pain severity or dysfunction.[12] Some patients experience pain over long periods of time yet life functioning is not changed in major ways. There are other patients with similar structural abnormalities who suffer substantially more and cannot maintain their usual levels of activity.[13] These patients may engage in behaviors that are maladaptive, amplify sensations, spend more time resting, and complain of less ability to control pain.[14,15]

Patients seek care from physical therapists, chiropractors, acupuncturists, or an ever-increasing number of other clinicians specializing in pain care. Despite professionals caring for pain problems and the development of specialists in pain management, most patients continue to rely on their primary care clinicians for pain control. When pain treatment from a specialist fails and the pain becomes part of daily living, patients return to primary care, where they have developed relationships built on trust, experience, and care for their entire family.

This book is designed to help primary care providers who deal with back and neck pain on a daily basis. The format of short chapters and bulleted highlights takes into account busy providers dealing with multiple complaints in a single patient. Primary care providers are capable of comprehensive evaluations and treatments; they understand complex pathophysiology and complicated family dynamics. Yet limited time requires an expedient approach. Cursory reviews and prioritizing care is more common. This book is designed to allow for quick treatment decisions but also provides a more complete review of back and neck pain. The topics range from pathophysiology, assessment, and comorbidity management to a variety of treatment options. With the current emphasis on opioid analgesia for persistent pain and the public health concern of prescription drug abuse, a chapter is devoted to safe opioid prescribing and making your practice environment safe while providing patient comfort.

Pain management has made tremendous advances in the last 15 years, yet much is written about the lack of knowledge and pain care deficiencies found in primary care. The authors understand the time pressure involved in the typical practice setting. This book is designed to help the busy primary care provider interested in compassionate, state-of-the-art pain management.

References

1. Jayson MI. Acute back pain. *Clin Med*. 2001;1:188–189.

2. Woolf AD, Pfleger B. Burden of major musculoskeletal conditions. *Bull World Health Org*. 2003;81:646–656.

3. National Institute of Neurological Disorders and Stroke. Pain: hope through research. 2009. Available at: http://www.ninds.nih.gov/disorders/chronic_pain/detail_chronic_pain.htm. Accessed May 24, 2011.

4. Lawrence RC, Felson DT, Helmick CG, et al. Estimates of the prevalence of arthritis and other rheumatic conditions in the United States. Part II. *Arthritis Rheum*. 2008;58:26–35.

5. Blount BW, Hart G, Ehreth JL. A description of the content of army family practice. *J Am Board Fam Pract*. 1993;6:143–152.

6. Raspe H, Hueppe A, Neuhauser H. Back pain, a communicable disease? *Int J Epidemiol*. 2008;37:69–74.

7. United States Bone and Joint Decade. The burden of musculoskeletal diseases. 2009. Available at: http://www.boneandjointburden.org. Accessed May 24, 2011.

8. Licciardone JC. The epidemiology and medical management of low back pain during ambulatory medical care visits in the United States. *Osteopath Med Prim Care*. 2008;2:11.

9. United States Bone and Joint Decade. The burden of musculoskeletal diseases. 2009. Available at: http://www.boneandjointburden.org. Accessed May 24, 2011.

10. Collins JJ BC, Sharda CE, Ozminkowski RJ, et al. The assessment of chronic health conditions on work performance, absence, and total economic impact for employers. *J Occup Environ Med*. 2005;47(6):547–557.

11. Kaiser Permanente. Controlling presenteeism. A healthy and productive workforce is the solution. 2009. Available at: http://www.kaiserinsuranceonline.com/pdf/presenteeismCA.pdf. Accessed May 24, 2011.

12. Flor H, Turk DC. Chronic back pain and rheumatoid arthritis: predicting pain and disability from cognitive variables. *J Behav Med*. 1988;11:251–265.

13. Sanders SH, Brena SF, Spier CJ, Beltrutti D, McConnell H, Quintero O. Chronic back pain patients around the world: cross-cultural similarities and differences. *Clin J Pain*. 1992;8:317–323.

14. Reesor KA, Craig KD. Medically incongruent chronic back pain physical limitations, suffering, and ineffective coping. *Pain*. 1988;32:35–45.

15. Pinsky J. Chronic pain syndromes and their treatment. In: Brodwin MG, Tellez F, Brodwin SK, eds. *Medical, Psychosocial and Vocational Aspects of Disability*. Athens, Ga: Elliott & Fitzpatrick, 1993:179–194.

Chapter 2

Pathophysiology

Steven Stanos

The International Association for the Study of Pain (IASP) describes pain as "an unpleasant sensory and emotional experience associated with actual or potential tissue damage, or described in terms of such damage." Pain is generally categorized as acute or chronic depending on the duration of symptoms as well as a person's physiologic response. Acute pain typically follows tissue injury, and it is brief in duration, reversible, and generally resolves with healing. Acute pain can be thought of as a "symptom" and only after a long term do consequences of nervous system activation lead to chronic pain, which is represented, assessed, and treated as a chronic disease.[1]

Neuropathic pain also differs significantly from acute nociceptive pain. In neuropathic pain, there are changes in the nervous system, which include changes in the peripheral tissue near the site of injury, more proximally along the primary and secondary neurons to the spinal cord (dorsal horn), and in the more ascending systems of the subcortical and cortical regions of the brain.

Nociceptive versus Neuropathic Pain

- Nociceptive pain
  - Believed to be related to ongoing activation of an intact nervous system by tissue injury
  - Somatic
  - Visceral
- Neuropathic pain
  - Believed to be related to aberrant somatosensory processing in the peripheral nervous system, the central nervous system, or both

Pain Theory

Overview

Hippocrates first hypothesized that four bodily fluids or humors were responsible for the state of one's personality, and any illness (physical or psychological) was responsible for pain. Seventeenth-century Renaissance thinking led to a more reductionist view of pain, separating "mind" from "body" and identifying more "specific" pathways responsible for the sensation of pain, and in many ways ignoring psychological influences.[2] The French philosopher Rene Descartes proposed a more biomedical sensory model for pain. Descartes' theory held that injury activates specific pain receptors and fibers that project pain impulses to a "pain center" in the brain. Pain experience was held to be proportional to peripheral injury. An understanding based on "specific" pathways of pain dominated the science of pain physiology until more comprehensive ones were developed in the twentieth century.

In 1965, Melzack and Wall proposed the gate control theory, representing an important advancement in understanding the complex biological and psychological aspects of pain sensation, experience, and behavior[3] Wall and Melzack's theory emphasized modulation of inputs in the spinal dorsal horn and the dynamic role of the spinal cord and brain in modulating (increasing or decreasing) pain inputs and outputs and thus the transmission of pain impulses and the perception of pain. The spinal cord is not just a passive conduit for pain transmission, but an active modulator of pain signals. Activity in large myelinated afferent fibers activates dorsal horn neurons that inhibit ascending transmission by secondary neurons and pathways to higher brain centers.

Melzack and Casey three years later emphasized motivational, affective, and cognitive aspects of the pain experience. Neural pathways could activate both sensory discriminative information about the location and intensity of pain, and more emotional and motivational effects of pain experience. Descending inhibition from cortical structures could also influence pain. Descending modulation of the "gate" theoretically could block nociceptive signals at the dorsal horn and provide the basis for behavioral induced reduction of pain. In turn, psychological processes, such as depression, could potentially increase pain by "opening" gating mechanisms at the dorsal horn. This modulation, carried down to the dorsal horn, provides a way for the central nervous system to actively modulate the afferent input at multiple levels of the central nervous system. This impacts all aspects of the pain experience, including affective, subjective, and evaluative components.

The gate control theory (See Figure 2.1) offered a new model for the successful integration of experimental and clinical observations related to the study of pain. Although challenged as somewhat incomplete, the theory has remained the core of contemporary pain science. It has spurred the development of new clinical treatments, including neurophysiologically based procedures (TENS, spinal cord stimulation), and pharmacologic, cognitive, and behavioral treatments. Primary care management can use this theory to help better understand the relationship connecting increased anxiety and depression with chronic pain, and on the treatment side, use deep breathing and other relaxation techniques to gate the pain at the brain and spinal cord. Pharmacologic approaches will also be used to modulate this gating system (i.e., increase monoamines [serotonin and norepinephrine], increase GABA, decrease substance P, glutamate, and other excitatory transmitters).

More recent understanding of pain physiology has better defined and elucidated the complex nature of how pain is perceived first as a peripheral trigger and the subsequent processes along the ascending and descending central nervous system and brain networks.

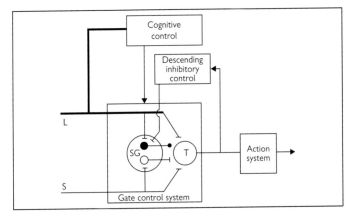

Figure 2.1 Gate control theory.

Neuromatrix

Melzack has extended the basic tenants of the gate control theory into an even more unified system described as the body-self neuromatrix. The neuromatrix includes the sensory, affective, and evaluative components of pain from the gate control theory, and it incorporates parallel inputs a person experiences over time. These include cognitive-related inputs (memories of past experiences, attention, anxiety, and meaning); sensory signaling stimuli (cutaneous, visceral, and musculoskeletal inputs); and resultant outputs from the brain network such as pain perception (sensory, affective, and cognitive dimensions), action responses (involuntary and voluntary), and stress-regulated changes (cortisol and other neurohumoral changes on the body) (See Figure 2.2).[4]

Pain Physiology

Overview

In a normal homeostatic state, cutaneous, visceral, and musculoskeletal pain serves as an alarm system to the body that indicates damage or potential damage in the environment. The purpose of nociception is to alert the organism to this potential damage so that avoidance behavior can be initiated. In contrast, chronic pain states may represent an alteration involving damage or injury to the central nervous system that serves no real protective role, reflecting a "pathologic" as opposed to "physiologic" state. Physiologic pain is initiated by specialized sensory "nociceptors" that innervate peripheral tissues, and which are activated by noxious stimuli (i.e., heat, mechanical), causing an inflow of action potentials ascending along neurons to the spinal cord and higher brain structures. This nociceptive input also activates reflex withdrawal, arousal, emotional, autonomic, and neurohumoral responses.[5]

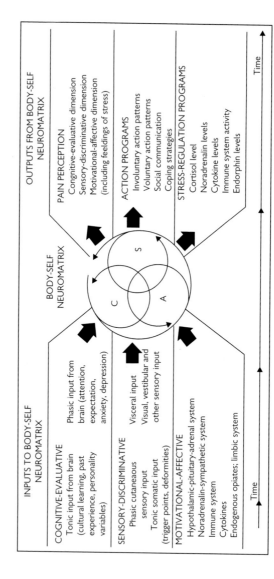

INPUTS TO BODY-SELF NEUROMATRIX

COGNITIVE-EVALUATIVE
Tonic input from brain
(cultural learning, past
experience, personality
variables)

Phasic input from
brain (attention,
expectation,
anxiety, depression)

SENSORY-DISCRIMINATIVE
Phasic cutaneaous
sensory input
Tonic somatic input
(trigger points, deformities)

Visceral input
Visual, vestibular and
other sensory input

MOTIVATIONAL-AFFECTIVE
Hypothalamic-pituitary-adrenal system
Noradrenalin-sympathetic system
Immune system
Cytokines
Endogenous opiates; limbic system

BODY-SELF NEUROMATRIX

C   S   A

OUTPUTS FROM BODY-SELF NEUROMATRIX

PAIN PERCEPTION
Congnitive-evaluative dimension
Sensory-discriminative dimension
Motivational-affective dimension
(including feeldings of stress)

ACTION PROGRAMS
Involuntary action patterns
Voluntary action patterns
Social communication
Coping strategies

STRESS-REGULATION PROGRAMS
Cortisol level
Noradrenalin levels
Cytokine levels
Immune system activity
Endorphin levels

Time

Time

Figure 2.2 Body-self neuromatrix. *Source:* Reprinted with permission from Melzack R. Pain and the neuromatrix in the brain. *J Dental Education.* 2001;65:1378–1382.

Primary Sensory Afferents

Mechanisms of normal peripheral sensation are critical in the development of chronic pain. A number of peripheral sensory afferent neurons with somata located among their respective dorsal root ganglia (i.e., cervical and lumbar) and cranial ganglia (i.e., face and head) respond to nonnoxious mechanical (mechanoreceptors), thermal (thermoreceptors), or chemical (chemoreceptors), and are associated with characteristic end structure receptors, thresholds for activation, and duration or response.[6]

Primary sensory afferents can be broadly defined by four types[7,8]:

1. Large-caliber, heavily myelinated muscle spindle and golgi tendon afferents that signal limb position and maintain proprioceptive sense
2. Large-caliber, heavily myelinated Aβ axons responsible for signaling highly discriminative mechanical stimuli
3. Small-caliber, lightly myelinated Aδ axons
4. Small, unmyelinated C axons that form free nerve endings that terminate in the epidermis, adjacent to vasculature, all around skin tissue, in visceral organs, and in bone

The complex interaction between the initial stimulus of tissue injury and the subjective experience of nociception and acute and/or chronic pain can be described by four general processes known as transduction, transmission, modulation, and perception. (See Table 2.1.)

Nociception: Transduction/Transmission/Modulation

Normal pain or "nociception" is characterized primarily by the processes of *transduction* and *transmission*, with minimal emphasis on modulation and a "normal" perception process. However, with chronic or persistent pain states, the process of *modulation* is more active, reflecting signal- and activity-dependent neuroplasticity and, in some cases, degeneration of peripheral and central nervous system structures. Finally, *perception* encompasses the subjective multidimensional individual processing from initial cortex activation through the final output of diverse neural networks responsible for the individual experience of

---

Table 2.1 **Signal Processing**

Transduction (receptor activation): One form of energy (thermal, mechanical, or chemical stimulus) is converted electrochemically into nerve impulses (action potentials) in primary afferents.

Transmission: Coded information is transferred from primary afferent fibers to spinal cord dorsal horn and onto brainstem, thalamus, and higher cortical structures.

Modulation: Activity- and signal-induced dorsal horn neural plasticity, which includes altered receptor and channel function (i.e., wind-up and central sensitization), gene expression, and changes in brain-mediated descending inhibition and facilitation.

Perception: Begins with activation of sensory cortex. The cortex is in intimate communication with motor and prefrontal cortex, which initiate efferent responses, as well as more primitive structures involved in the emotive aspects of pain.

Source: Wolf CJ, Costigan M. Transcriptional and posttranslational plasticity and the generation of inflammation. *Proc Natl Acad Sci USA.* 1999;96:7723–7730.

pain and pain-related suffering. These four general processes are reviewed next and serve as an important foundation for more clearly understanding complex pain mechanisms, and possible rational pharmacotherapeutic interventional and cognitive-behavioral treatment approaches.

Transduction

The principal receptors for pain are the branched endings of C and Aδ fibers in the skin, muscles, and joints. Damaging (or potentially damaging) energy in the cellular environment impacts the free nerve endings, and the complicated cellular processes of nociceptive transduction occur. Inflammatory cascades are concurrently activated (prostaglandin, leukotriene, etc.) and immediately become principal players in the transduction process. Recent histochemical studies have revealed two broad categories of C fibers: peptidergic and lectin IB4 (isolectin B$_4$) binding. Peptidergic fibers contain a variety of the peptide neurotransmitters, including substance P (SP) and calcitonin gene-related peptide (CGRP), and express tyrosine receptor kinase A (trkA) receptors, which show high affinity for nerve growth factors (NGFs). Peptidergic neurons appear to be key players in neurogenic inflammation (where the transduction cells themselves become active participants in the local inflammatory process) and other chronic inflammatory states.[9,10] The other class, IB$_4$, contains few neuropeptides, but it expresses a surface carbohydrate group selectivity binding to the plant lectin IB$_4$ and is supported by glial-derived neurotrophic factor.[11] IB$_4$ expresses P2X3 receptors, a subtype of ATP-gated ion channels.[12] Differences in supporting trophic factors might be responsible for differing functional responses to painful stimuli between these distinct C-fiber types.

There are probably multiple arachodonic acid residue receptors involved (prostaglandin, leucotriene, etc.), and the "chaos" level of complexity is further complicated by the very active presence of the support cells (glia and myelin) and the efferent input by the central nervous system itself, primarily via the sympathetic nervous system. There are noradrenergic receptors on the transduction cell, and these can be "uncovered" or activated in inflamed tissue.

Aδ nociceptors (also responders to noxious, thermal, and chemical stimuli) are most easily classified on functional grounds. Type II exhibit short response latencies to heat and are activated at relatively higher thresholds (43C). Type II Aδ are responsible for the initial sensation of a burn stimulus. Type I Aδ exhibit longer response latencies and are activated at much higher temperatures (>50°C).[13] Type I Aδ and nociceptive C fibers are more commonly associated with persistent painful sensations.

Transmission

Cutaneous peripheral afferent neurons can be classified into three types based on diameter, structure, and conduction velocity of action potentials. In general, C fibers (thin, unmyelinated, slowly conducting, 0.5–2.0 m sec^{-1}), Aδ (medium, thinly myelinated, rapidly conducting, 12–30 m sec^{-1}) carry noxious stimuli, and Aβ fibers (large, myelinated and fast, 30–100 m sec^{-1}) carry innocuous stimuli (touch, vibration, and pressure) (see Fig. 2.3) except in situations of peripheral or central sensitization. The percentage of distribution of nociceptors in the skin is roughly proportioned 70%, 10%, and 20%, respectively. With peripheral and central neuroplastic changes in Aβ fibers, innocuous stimuli might be

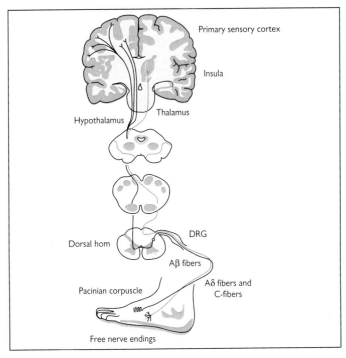

Figure 2.3 The neural loop. *Source:* Reprinted with permission from Argoff CD, Abrecht P, Irving G, Rice F. Multimodal analgesia for chronic pain: rationale and future directions. *Pain Med.* 2009;10:S53–66.

perceived as painful, resulting in allodynia. Aδ nociceptors respond to intense mechanical and temperature stimuli and with sensitization contribute to the process called hyperpathia (where noxious stimuli becomes frankly more painful, and the pain perception can last even after the initial stimuli is removed). Most C fibers are polymodal transducers. Aß fibers demonstrate encapsulated nerve endings involved in non-nociceptive function. Aδ fibers mediate the fast, prickling quality of pain, whereas C fibers mediate the slow, burning quality of pain. An additional class of nociceptors, the so-called silent or sleeping nociceptors, make up approximately 10%–20% of C fibers in the skin, joints, and viscera and are normally unresponsive to acute noxious stimuli. With inflammation and tissue injury, these "silent" nociceptors are sensitized via activation of second-messenger systems and the release of a number of local chemical mediators (i.e., bradykinin, prostaglandins, serotonin, and histamine) and may contribute to temporal and spatial summation, increasing afferent input at the dorsal horn.[14,15]

Modulation
Primary afferents subserving distinct input from cutaneous, muscle, and visceral tissues converge at the dorsal horn. Several ascending pathways are involved

in transferring and modulating this nociceptive input. At the cellular level, the influx of sodium is fundamental to electrical signaling and subsequent generation of action potentials and excitatory postsynaptic potentials. This is followed by calcium channel opening, contributing to more prolonged depolarization as well as second-messenger molecular changes, involved in more permanent neuroplastic central nervous system changes. At the synaptic terminal of the axon, action potentials lead to the release of neurotransmitters. Neurotransmitter release is dependent on specific ion channels. Ion channels are either *ligand gated*, opening in response to binding of ligands to receptors, or *voltage gated*, opening in response to changes in membrane potentials.[16] Other targeted receptor and ion channels include vanilloid or TRPV-1(capsaicin) receptor, heat-activated, ATP-gated purinergeic receptor (P2X), proton-gated or acid-sensing ion channels (ASIC), and voltage-gated Na channels. The vanilloid receptor is a nonselective cation channel (TRPV-1) activated by elevated temperature (>43°C) and acidification.

Aδ and C fibers convey nociceptive information primarily to superficial laminae (I/II) and deep laminae (V/VI) of the dorsal horn. Lamina I plays an important role in relaying information on the current state of tissues, including damaging mechanical stress, heat and cold, local metabolism (acid pH, hypoxia), cell breakdown (ATP, glutamate), mast cell activation (serotonin and bradykinin), and immune activity (cytokines).[17] Aβ fibers transmit innocuous, mechanical stimuli to deeper laminae (III–VI). Lamina I cells are activated by nociceptive-specific (NS) neurons, whereas lamina V cells respond to a wide dynamic range (WDR) neurons of "wide" stimulus intensities. WDR neurons receive input from mechanoreceptive Aβ fibers and nociceptive (Aδ and C) fibers.

Normal synaptic transmission conduction of action potentials at the dorsal horn initiates neurotransmitter release. Low-intensity stimulations (i.e., brush, touch, or vibration) activate Aβ fibers only, releasing fast glutamate-mediated postsynaptic currents. Fast excitatory glutamate transmission is co-released presynaptically with the neuropeptides such as substance P (SP), CGRP, cholecystokinin (CCK), proteins (BDNF), and glial-derived factors.[18] Glutamate acts on a range of transmission cell receptors such as NMDA (slow current), AMPA (fast current) glutamate receptors, and gated ion channels. With normal transmission, calcium flows only through the AMPA receptor, while the NMDA receptor is blocked by magnesium, depolarizing the cell and leading to a proportional response. Prolonged depolarization of the postsynaptic cell causes voltage-dependent magnesium removal, opening the channel, allowing additional sodium and calcium to enter the cell. This amplified evoked response to subsequent input describes the process of "windup."[19]

Ascending and Descending Modulation

Melzack and Casey's classic descriptions of neuroanatomical pathways make a distinction between the lateral and medial pain systems corresponding to their relationship with the thalamus.[20] The two systems are highly interdependent, the lateral (neo-spinothalamic) system, generally representing sensory-discriminative dimensions, versus the medial (paleospinothalamic) system involving more motivational-affective and cognitive-evaluative dimensions of the pain experience. Additional ascending pathways, including the spinothalamic, spinomesencephalic, spinoreticular, spinolimbic, spinocervical, and dorsal column pathways, are described elsewhere.[21]

The lateral system projects to the ventral posterolateral and ventral posteromedial thalamic nuclei prior to projecting to the somatosensory and premotor cortices. The motor input is nearly as large as the sensory input, and this theoretically prepares the recipient of the painful input for the appropriate efferent (behavioral) response. The more medial pathway projects to the medial thalamic nuclei and limbic cortices, which include the anterior cingulated cortex (ACC), orbitofrontal cortex, and amygdala. The medial system involves important connections with periaqueductal gray (PAG), a key area involved in modulating nociceptive inhibition and behavioral responses to potentially threatening stimuli.[22] Animal and human studies have identified the ACC in regulating avoidance behaviors and the perception of pain unpleasantness.[23] Only a small portion of these action potentials normally reach the thalamus and higher brain centers because of significant modulating or filtering effects at the spinal cord and brainstem. Of course, with prolonged pathology and inflammation these filters "break down," contributing to central sensitization.

Endogenous Pain Systems

In addition to descending inhibition, the endogenous inhibitory system also includes local endogenous opioids (from peri-aqueductal gray), biogenic amines (serotonin and neropeniphrine), and γ-aminobutyric acid (GABA), which generally act to inhibit pain signals. Important excitatory transmitters in this system include glutamate and substance P.[24,25] Besides descending inhibition from cortical areas, recent studies have suggested descending facilitatory pathways may link brainstem and spinal cord areas via pronociceptive serotonergic and opioid mechanisms.[26,27] These pronociceptive pathways may help explain possible mechanisms of persistent pain signs and symptoms, such as allodynia and hyperalgesia, that are common to chronic pain conditions.[28]

Pathways originating from the spinal cord dorsal horn activate brain structures involved in rudimentary aspects of autonomic system response (i.e., escape, arousal, and fear), including the medulla and midbrain reticular formation, amygdale, hypothalamus, and thalamic nuclei.[29] Activation of somatosensory cortices (S1S2) provides information regarding the quality and intensity of pain.[30] Affective aspects of the pain experience, such as pain unpleasantness, reflect more of the aversive qualities of the pain experience, such as the "suffering" component.

Higher processing involves parietal and insular regions, contributing to an overall sense of intrusion and unpleasantness.[31] Finally, convergence of these pathways with more frontal regions, such as anterior cingulate cortex (ACC), is responsible for attention and "emotional valence" of the overall pain experience.

Although cutaneous and visceral pain share common cortical and subcortical networks, differences in response pattern, frequency, and processing might underlie differences in quality, affect, and resultant behavioral responses[32]

Visceral pain has a more indistinct quality, poor localization, and in general, is associated with autonomic markers such as bradycardia and hypotension. Cutaneous nociceptive reactions more classically involve protective reflexes such as tachycardia and hypertension.

Brian Processing of Pain[33]

Brain imaging studies indicate both cortical and subcortical areas are important in the complex experience of pain and pain-related suffering (See Figure 2.4). Neuromiaging studies have identified a network of somatosensory, limbic, and associated structures (frontal cortex), all of which act with parallel inputs from multiple nociceptive pathways. Somatosensory and discriminatory function of pain may include S2 and insular cortex (IC) and more affective and motivational aspects of pain involving the cingulated cortex. Different pain states and conditions may alter their affect on brain modulation. Pain Matrix

- Anterior cingulate cortex (ACC)
  - Both primary somatosensory cortex (S1) and secondary somatosensory cortex (S2) are activated in heat pain studies.
  - Anterior cingulated (ACC) and insular (IC) cortices are activated during many painful stimuli and are implicated in affective processing of pain.[34]
  - Important subcortical regions include the thalamus, basal ganglia, and cerebellum.
- Insular cortex (IC)
- Thalamus
- Sensorimotor cortex (SSI, SSII)
- Cerebellum

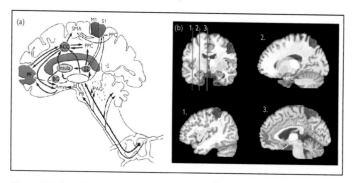

Figure 2.4 Cortical and subcortical regions involved in pain perception, their interconnectivity and ascending pathways. (*a*) Schematic shows the regions, their interconnectivity and afferent pathways. (*b*) The areas corresponding to those shown in the schematic are shown in an anatomical magnetic resonance image, on a coronal slice and three saggital slices as indicated on the coronal slice. *Source:* Reprinted from Apkarian AV, Bushnell MC, Treede R, Zubieta J. Human brain mechanisms of pain perception and regulation in health and disease.[33] *Eur J Pain.* 2005;9(4):63–84, with permission from Elsevier.

Peripheral Sensitization

C fibers and Aδ receptors undergo changes in response to tissue injury such as inflammation, ischemia, and compression. These changes are marked at the peripheral terminals by the release of chemical mediators from damaged and inflammatory cells (See Figure 2.5). The so-called inflammatory soup, rich in algesic substances, causes a lowering of threshold for activation and subsequent evoked pain. Algogenic substances also activate second-messenger systems, which induce gene expression in the cell. Excitatory amino acids and neuropeptides (SP, CGRP, and neurokinins) are released by peripheral and central nociceptive C fibers, inducing neurogenic inflammation. Neurogenic inflammation involves retrograde release of algogenic substances, which in turn excites other nearby nociceptors, creating local feed-forward loops of sensitization and activation. Peripheral sensitization leads to changes locally at the skin or cutaneous level but may serve as an ongoing drive of aberrant activity to the dorsal horn and in turn contribute to more persistent and chronic neuroplastic changes in the central nervous system, characterized by central sensitization.

Central Sensitization

"Central sensitization" describes a complex set of activation-dependent post-translational changes occurring at the dorsal horn, brainstem, and higher cerebral sites. Sensitization involves facilitation of pain transmission after injury. Input from peripheral tissues and nociceptors generate long-term potentiation at the dorsal horn. Presynaptically, release of excitatory neurotransmitters (glutamate, substance P, and brain-derived neurotrophic factor [BDNF]) results in changes in activation of related receptors and channels (as described earlier). This results in an increase in calcium influx and resultant depolarization (and efflux from cytoplasmic organelles), contributing to potentiation of the cell by activation of calcium-dependent enzymes protein kinases (protein

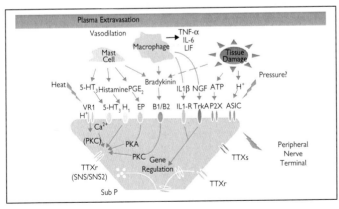

Figure 2.5 Peripheral sensitization. *Source:* Adapted from Woolf CJ, et al. Neuronal plasticity, increasing the gain in pain. *Science.* 2000;288:1765–1768.

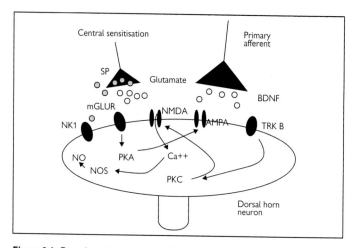

Figure 2.6 Central sensitization. *Source:* Reprinted with permission from Jensen TS, Gottrup H, Kasch H, et al. Has basic research contributed to chronic pain treatment? *Acta Anaesthesiol Scand.* 2001;45:1128–1135.

Table 2.2 **Mechanisms of Nociceptive Central Pain**
1. Autosensitization of receptors
2. Ectopic firing of DRG cells
3. Calcium-induced molecular cascades from excess glutamate
4. Phenotypic change of Aβ cells and DRG
5. Changes in gene expression of sodium channels and neuropeptides
6. Anatomic changes at dorsal horn

Source: Schwarzman RJ, Grothusen J, Kiefer TR, Rohr P. Neuropathic central pain. *Arch Neurol.* 2001;58:1547–1550.

kinase C [PKC], cyclic adenosine 3,5 monophosphate [cAMP] and tRK).[35] Posttranslational changes also include phosphorylation of NMDA and AMPA receptors, activation of second messengers such as nitric-oxide (NO), and central prostaglandin production,[36] resulting in upregulation of the cell and neuronal hyperexcitability (See Figure 2.6 and Table 2.2).

References

1. Carr D, Goudas L. Acute pain. *Lancet.* 1999;353:2051–2057.
2. Descarte R, De Homine. Leiden, Netherlands: Moyardus and Leffen; 1662.
3. Melzack R, Wall P. Pain mechanisms: a new theory. *Science.* 1965;150:971–979.

4. Melzack R. Evolution of the neuromatrix theory of pain. The Prithivi Raj Lecture. Paper presented at: The Third World Congress of World Institute of Pain; Month 2004; Barcelona. *Pain Practice* 2005;5:85–94.

5. Woolf CJ, Slater MW. Neuronal plasticity, increasing the gain in pain. *Science.* 2000;288:1765–1768.

6. Raja S, Meyer R, Ringkamp M, Campbell J. Peripheral neural mechanisms of nociception. In: Wall P, Melzack R, eds. *Textbook of Pain.* London: Harcourt; 1999:11–57.

7. Kidd B, Urban L. Mechanisms of inflammatory pain. *Br J Anaesth.* 2001;87:3–11.

8. Millan J. Induction of pain: an integrative review. *Prog Neurobiol.* 1999;57:1–164.

9. Cao Y, Mantyh P, Carlson E. Primary afferent tachykinins are required to experience moderate to severe pain. *Nature.* 1998;392:390–394.

10. Woolf CJ, Mannion R, Neumann S. Null mutations lacking substance: elucidating pain mechanisms by genetic pharmacology. *Neuron.* 1998;20:1063–1066.

11. Stucky C, Gold M, Ahan X. Mechanisms of pain. *Proc Natl Acad Sci USA.* 2001;98(21):11845–11846.

12. Julius D, Basbaum JA. Molecular mechanisms of nociception. *Nature.* 2001;413:203–210.

13. Caterina M, Julius D. Sense and specificity: a molecular identity for nociceptors. *Curr Opin Neurobiol.* 1999;9:525–530.

14. Schaible H, Schmidt R. Time course of mechanosensitivity changes in articular afferents during a developing experimental arthritis. *J Neurophysiol.* 1988;60:2190–2195.

15. Cervero F. Sensory innervation of the viscera: peripheral basis of visceral pain. *Physiol Rev.* 1994;74:95–138.

16. Sadock BJ, Sadock VA. The brain and behavior. In: Sadock BJ, Kaplan HI, Sadock VA, eds. *Kaplan and Sadock's Synopsis of Psychiatry.* 9th edn. Philadelphia, Pa: Lippincott Williams & Wilkins; 2003:72–78.

17. Craig AD. Pain mechanisms: labeled lines versus convergence in central processing. *Ann Rev Neurosci.* 2003;26:1–30.

18. Mannion RJ, Woolf C. Pain mechanisms and management: a central perspective. *Clin J Pain.* 2000;16:S144-S156.

19. Mannion RJ, Woolf CJ. Pain mechanisms and management: a central perspective. *Clin J Pain.* 2000;16:S144-S156.

20. Melzack R, Casey K. Sensory, motivational and central control determinants of pain: a new conceptual model. In: Kenshalo D, ed. *The Skin Senses.* Springfield, Ill: Thomas; 966:423–443.

21. Willis WD, Westlund KN. Neuroanatomy of the pain system and of the pathways that modulate pain. *J Clin Neurophysiol.* 1997;14:2–31.

22. Nicholson K, Martelli M. The problem of pain. *J Head Trauma Rehabil.* 2004;19:2–9.

23. Koyana T, Kato K, Mikami A. During pain-avoidance neurons activated in the macaque anterior cingulated and caudate. *Neurosci Lett.* 2000;283:17–20.

24. Kidd B, Urban L. Mechanisms of inflammatory pain. *Br J Anaesth.* 2001;87:3–11.

25. Woolf CJ. Pain: moving from symptom control toward mechanisms-specific pharmacologic management. *Ann Intern Med.* 2004;140:441–451.

26. Suzuki R, Rygh LJ, Dickenson AH. Bad news from the brain: descending 5-HT pathways that control spinal pain processing. *Trends Pharmacol Sci.* 2004;25(12):613–617.

27. Fields H. State-dependent opiod control of pain. *Nat Rev Neurosci.* 2004;5:565–575.

28. Porreca F, Ossipov MH, Gebhart GF. Chronic pain and medullary descending facilitation. *Trends Neurosci.* 2002;25(6):319–325.

29. Price D. Psychological and neural mechanisms of the affective dimension of pain. *Science.* 2000;288:1769–1772.

30. Hofbauer R, Rainville P, Duncan G, et al. Cortical representation of the sensory dimension of pain. *J Neurophysiol.* 2001;86:402–411.

31. Rainville P, Duncan G, Price D, et al. Pain affect encoded in human anterior cingulated but not somatosensory cortex. *Science.* 1997;277:968–971.

32. Strigo I, Duncan G, Boivin M, et al. Differentiation of visceral and cutaneous pain in the human brain. *J Neurophysiol.* 2003;89:3294–3303.

33. Apkarian V, Bushnell MC, Treede R, Zubieta JK. Human brain mechanisms of pain perception and regulation in health and disease. *Eur J Pain.* 2005;9:463–484.

34. Rainville P, Duncan G, Price D, et al. Pain affect encoded in human anterior cingulated but not somatosensory cortex. *Science.* 1997;277:968–971.

35. Malenka R, Nicol R. Long-term potentiation- a decade of progress. *Science.* 1999;285(5435):1870–1874.

36. Woolf C, Costigan M. Transcriptional and posttranslational plasticity and the generation of inflammatory pain. *Proc Natl Acad Sci USA.* 1999;96:7723–7730.

Chapter 3

Evaluation and Diagnosis

Yvonne D'Arcy

The evaluation and diagnosis of patients with low back pain and neck pain can be difficult and often inconclusive. For patients with low back pain, the results of scanning and radiographic studies may be negative while the pain persists. This can be the result of soft tissue injury, which can be highly painful yet more subjective and relies on the patient's self-report of pain. Neck pain from a whiplash injury may fall into the same category: extremely painful, but with very little definitive evidence to make a firm diagnosis.

Pain Assessment

The key to providing adequate treatment for a patient with back or neck pain, acute or chronic, is to do a thorough evaluation and assessment of the pain. For acute pain a numeric pain intensity rating may be adequate, but for chronic back or neck pain, a more complete assessment is needed. For the patient whose pain is in the acute stage, using the Numeric Rating Scale (NRS) with a 0 to 10 pain rating may be adequate. If the patient can achieve a 2-point decrease on the NRS or a 30% reduction in intensity, the decrease is considered to be clinically significant.[1] What these numeric decreases are best at measuring is really the efficacy of the medication or intervention being used to treat the pain.

For patients with chronic pain, a more formal comprehensive pain assessment tools such as the Brief Pain Inventory (BPI), the McGill Pain Questionnaire (MPQ), or a combination of the two may provide better insight into the pain being experienced by the patient. These tools are reliable and valid and include body diagrams, NRS, pain descriptors, functionality questions, and questions about medication efficacy.

One technique for assessing chronic pain that is helpful for the busy practitioner is to use a standardized set of interview questions that will address most aspects of the pain complaint and provide additional history about the patient's use of pain management strategies. The Brief Pain Impact Questionnaire (Table 3.1) is designed for use by a practitioner who is completing a full or first-time pain assessment.

For most patients, using the 4 A's of assessment and reassessment will provide adequate information on the success of the selected pain regimen.

- **A**ssessment/reassessment of pain intensity
- **A**ctivity: How has it improved?

Table 3.1 Brief Pain Impact Questionnaire

- How strong is your pain, right now, worst/average over the past week?
- How many days over the past week have you been unable to do what you would like to do because of your pain?
- Over the past week, how often has pain interfered with your ability to take care of yourself, for example, with bathing, eating, dressing, and going to the toilet?
- Over the past week, how often has pain interfered with your ability to take care of your home-related chores such as grocery shopping, preparing meals, paying bills, and driving?
- How often do you participate in pleasurable activities such as hobbies, socializing with friends, and travel? Over the past week how often has pain interfered with these activities?
- How often do you do some type of exercise? Over the past week, how often has pain interfered with your ability to exercise?
- Does pain interfere with your ability to think clearly?
- Does pain interfere with your appetite? Have you lost weight?
- Does pain interfere with your sleep? How often over the last week?
- Has pain interfered with your energy, mood, personality, or relationships with other people?
- Over the past week have you taken pain medications?
- Has your use of alcohol or other drugs ever caused a problem for you or those close to you?
- How would you rate your health at the present time?

Source: Reprinted with permission from Weiner DK, Herr K, Rudy TE. *Persistent Pain in Older Adults: An Interdisciplinary Guide for Treatment.* New York, NY: Springer; 2003.

- **A**nalgesic efficacy: Are the pain medications providing the expected relief? Are there any side effects preventing you from using the medications for effective pain relief?
- **A**berrant behaviors: If opioid medication is involved, has the patient developed behaviors that indicate he or she is having problems controlling opioid use?

What are aberrant behaviors? Some patients who are taking opioids regularly to manage pain may develop behaviors that may be perceived as representing addiction. A patient may have behaviors that are outside of normal behavior, but are considered by many practitioners as a sign of addiction.

Some behaviors that are less predictive of addiction include the following: hoarding medications, taking someone else's medication, requesting a specific drug or dose, raising drug doses without a prescription several times, drinking more alcohol when in pain, smoking cigarettes to relieve pain, and using opioids to treat other symptoms. These behaviors may indicate unrelieved pain or the patient's inability to afford the medication that is prescribed to treat the pain.

There are some behaviors that are more concerning and may indicate addiction. Behaviors that are more predictive of addiction include concurrent use of illicit drugs, stealing or selling prescription drugs, injecting oral medications, repeated resistance to changes in therapy although there are clear negative effects, and deterioration in family and work relationships related to drug use.[2]

More information on opioid use and addiction will be provided in the safe prescribing chapter.

Basic Elements of a Pain Assessment for Verbal Patients

Location

Have the patient point to the area on the body that is painful. For multiple painful areas, have the patient locate each one individually. If one area is more painful than the next, make sure the most painful area is clearly identified. If there is a radiation of pain, for example, down a leg or arm, make sure the area is clearly defined so that the correct treatment options can be determined. For the patient with low back pain, pain that radiates down the sciatic nerve at the back of the leg may require a particular type of medication, an antidepressant or antiepileptic medication, or may indicate that an interventional option would be effective. A body diagram can be helpful when the patient is trying to locate the pain (see Fig. 3.1).

Duration

Ask the patient, "When did you first feel this pain?" and "How long does the pain last?" Explore any potential sources or causes of the pain. Ask whether the pain intensity varies during different times of the day and how long the periods of higher intensity pain last.

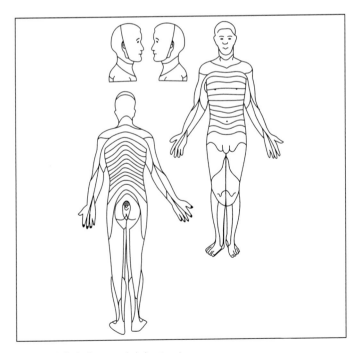

Figure 3.1 Body diagram to help locate pain.

Intensity

Use the NRS to have the patient rate the intensity of the pain. If there are times of the day or night when the pain intensity is more or less severe, ask whether the prescribed medication reduces the intensity of the pain. If the patient is taking pain medication, determine how effective the patient feels it is in decreasing the pain intensity.

Quality/Description

Have the patient describe the quality of the pain. This may be one of the most important items in the assessment process. If the patient uses words like *burning*, *tingling*, or *painful numbness*, it may indicate a neuropathic source for the pain.

Alleviating/Aggravating Factors

Most patients have some form of home treatment for pain and they most often will attempt to treat their pain before they seek health care.. If the patient has tried some form of pain relief, ask whether it helped, and whether it made the pain better or worse. Ask the patient whether activity made the pain worse or whether rest improved the pain. Ask the patient whether any one position is better than others for relieving the pain.

Pain Management Goal

For most patients with chronic pain, the concept of being pain-free is not a valid goal. Because of injury or continued pain from physiologic causes, the potential for ever removing all the pain is very low. Work with the patient to set a goal that is reasonable and achievable. Most patients with chronic pain have a pain intensity rating that will allow them to function at their highest level. Ask the patient what pain intensity he or she thinks is acceptable and then tailor pain interventions to achieve the patient's expectations. Consistent pain reassessment will track progress toward the goal that has been set.

Function Goal

Pain is dynamic and increases with activity.[3] Ask the patient how the pain interferes with his or her activities of daily living. Assess the patient for sleep disturbances that can affect the patient's ability to function. By setting a functionality goal, progress can be tracked at each subsequent visit.

Including the patient with chronic pain in the assessment process gives the patient a feeling of validation and encourages him or her to work toward the pain and functional goal. Providing maximum pain relief and functionality is the goal of any pain relief treatment for a chronic pain patient.[4,5,6,7]

Evaluation of Back and Neck Injuries

The evaluation of back and neck injuries includes a variety of physical assessments. After getting the full assessment of the pain complaint, the physical assessment and evaluation of the painful area will provide more information about the location and extent of the physical complaint.

Back Injuries

The evaluation and assessment of a back injury starts with the physical examination of the patient. Back pain may be caused by a variety of injuries or degenerative conditions Observing the patient's back for any signs of deformity and irregularity is the first step. Palpation along the spine is the easiest way to determine whether there are painful areas on the back. Herniated discs in the L5-S1 or L4-L5 vertebrae may produce tenderness at one or more of the following:

- Spinous processes
- Intervertebral joints
- Paravertebral muscles
- Sacrocaiatic notch
- Sciatic nerve

Rheumatoid arthritis may also be the cause of tenderness at the intervertebral joints.[8]

The American Pain Society and the American College of Physicians developed a joint guideline for diagnosing and treating low back pain. Guideline recommendations include a focused history and physical that indicates the frequency of symptoms, location and duration of the pain, history of the pain, and prior treatment.[9] Information on infection or neurologic symptoms such as muscle weakness is considered necessary.

For low back pain, the physical examination should include a straight leg raise test to assess for disc herniation. To perform this test, the patient lies on the examination table and raises his or her leg to a 30- to 70-degree angle. If pain is experienced, the test is positive for disc herniation or compression on the nerve route.[8] Using this test along with a neurologic exam that includes great toe dorsiflexion, plantar dorsiflexion, and ankle reflexes can help identify the area of pain.[9]

A further recommendation of the Guideline is that practitioners should try to avoid imaging or other diagnostic tests for patients with nonspecific back pain. This recommendation is related to the need to minimize unnecessary radiation exposure to the lumbar and lower abdominal area of the body.[9] Furthermore, using plain radiography with computed tomography (CT) or magnetic resonance imaging (MRI) as diagnostic techniques have not been associated with improved outcomes. If imaging is done, the recommendation is to use MRI because there is better visualization of the spinal structures. CT should be used only if the patient is a candidate for surgery or epidural steroid injection.[9]

Instances where imaging is recommended:

- Severe or progressive neurologic deficits
- A serious underlying condition
- Persistent low back pain and signs and symptoms of radiculopathy
- Suspected spinal stenosis
- Cancer with cord compression
- Vertebral infection
- Cauda equina syndrome

Neck Pain

Assessing and evaluating neck pain is similar to low back assessment. Palpation of the spinal processes for pain or muscle spasm is the first step. Neck flexion, extension, rotation, and lateral bending should be performed and any pain or radiation of pain should be noted. If there is tenderness or limited mobility of the neck, a full neurologic assessment should be performed.

Local muscle tenderness with pain on movement and no neurologic deficits indicates a mechanical neck pain. Pain from a whiplash injury will present with localized paracervical tenderness, decreased range of motion, and perceived weakness of the upper extremities.[8] Both of these conditions will respond to the usual medication and physical therapy regimens.

Patients who complain of sharp or burning pain in one arm with associated paresethesia and weakness have cervical nerve root compression resulting in cervical radiculopathy. Cervical myelopathy can be caused by a cervical cord compression. These patients will complain of neck pain with bilateral weakness and paresthesia in both upper and lower extremities, urinary frequency, hand clumsiness, palmar paresthesia, and gait changes. Neck flexion will exacerbate symptoms.[8] There may also be positive Babinski signs and Lhermitte sign (neck flexion causing an electrical shock sensation to radiate down the spine). Confirmation of cervical myelopathy indicates a need for a full neurologic evaluation.

Red Flags

Some acute low back pain may be the result of kidney or urinary tract infections that can be treated with antibiotics. Women who present with low back pain should also be evaluated for pelvic pathology, including ovarian cancer in appropriate patients. Infections are simpler to treat than other conditions with the same presentation.

Patients who complain of significant unintentional weight loss or pain that worsens at night and does not resolve with rest should be evaluated for the presence of a malignancy. Neurologic symptoms such as bowel and bladder dysfunction or foot drop accompanied by intense low back pain can signal a spinal cord compression or a neurologic disease. Progressive weakening in the lower extremities can indicate a cauda equine syndrome. All of these conditions are very serious and require a full evaluation.[10]

It is important to use the four A's to reassess the patient's condition at every clinic visit. Individualizing the patient's therapy will provide the best chance for positive outcomes. Reassessment can determine whether the selected therapy is working and will allow the health care provider to adjust medications and other therapeutics so that a steady progression toward increased functionality can be maintained.

A final consideration is the legal status of any patient. If the patient has an injury that is work- or accident-related, it is important to know what type of legal proceedings the patient is engaged in. If the patient's settlement depends on the prognosis, assessment, and reassessment for the injury, it is important that the health care provider do complete assessments and document the findings if they are to be used in court.

References

1 Farrar JT, Young JP, Lamoreaux L, Werth JL, Poole R. Clinical importantce of changes in chronic pain intensity measured on an 11 point numerical pain rating scale. *Pain*. 2001:94:149–158.

2 Fine P, Portnoy R. *Opioid Analgesia*. New York, NY: Vendome Group; 2007.

3 Dahl JB, Kehlet H. Postoperative pain and its management. In: McMahon SB, Kolzenburg M, eds. *Wall & Melzack's Textbook of Pain*. 5th ed. Philadelphia, Pa: Churchill Livingstone; 2006:100–126.

4 D'Arcy Y. *Compact Clinical Guide to Chronic Pain*. New York, NY: Springer Publications; 2010.

5 D'Arcy Y. Taking care of patients with low back pain using evidence based options. *Nurse Practitioner Journal*. 2009;9:17–18.

6 D'Arcy Y. Pain assessment. In: *Core Curriculum for Pain Management Nursing*. Dubuque, Iowa: Kendall Hunt; 2009:217–234.

7 D'Arcy YM. Pain assessment and management. In: Iyer PW, Levin BJ, Shea MA, eds. *Medical Legal Aspects of Medical Records*. Tucson, Ariz: Lawyers and Judges Publishing Co.; 2006:605–637.

8 Bickley L, Szilagyi P. *Bates Guide to Physical Assessment*. Philadelphia, Pa: Wolter Kluwer; 2009.

9 Chou R, Qaseem A, Snow V, et al. Diagnosis and treatment of low back pain: a joint clinical practice guideline from the American College of Physicians and the American Pain Society. *Ann Intern Med*. 2007;147(7):478–491.

10 D'Arcy Y. *Pain Management: Evidence-Based Tools and Techniques for Nursing Professionals*. Marblehead, Mass: HcPro; 2007.

Chapter 4

Physical Exam: Cervical and Lumbar Pain

Steven Stanos, Anjum Sayyad

A comprehensive pain examination includes a complete examination of the painful area, including bony structures, cartilage, joints, ligaments, tendons, bursa, nerves, and skin. A comprehensive examination for neck- and spine-related conditions includes a focused assessment of posture, core strength, balance, and gait. The exam findings will help the clinicians identify single or multiple causes for pain, compensatory changes that may also be present in chronic pain, both of which will be subsequently targeted by active and passive therapy approaches (i.e., modalities, physical therapy exercises).

The following sections will describe important aspects of a global pain assessment, and how the findings of this examination can help guide treatment. Key components of the physical exam include the following: posture, motor strength, muscle stretch reflexes, cervical and lumbar range of motion (ROM), provocative testing (i.e., facet, sacroiliac joint), dural tension (i.e., straight leg raise, slump seated), myofascial or soft tissue assessment, and pain behavior.

Overview of Comprehensive Physical Exam for Cervical and Lumbar Pain Conditions

- Posture
- Motor strength
- Sensory exam
- Muscle stretch reflexes (formerly referred to as deep tendon reflexes)
- Provocative testing
- Dural tension testing (i.e., nerve root signs)
- Sacroiliac joint testing
- Soft tissue and myofascial assessment
- Balance and gait
- Pain behavior

Posture/Standing Exam

Posture has been defined as "the position of the body at one point in time" and has a close relationship with position and function of related joints of the body.

A more "proper" posture may include when the joints of the body are aligned to create the least amount of stress and optimal muscle activation and balance. Abnormal posture promotes altered stresses on joints and causes mechanical dysfunction leading to pain and tissue damage. A study of elderly females found that prolonged flexed posture correlated with vertebral pain, muscle strength impairment, and disability.[1]

Posture may be observed indirectly during the patient interview or formally during the physical exam. In standing, normal posture includes cervical and lumbar lordosis and a slight thoracic kyphosis. Also assess the position of the head in relation to the shoulders as well as more global side-to-side asymmetries (i.e., right shoulder positioned superiorly, left iliac crest superior due to pelvic obliquity and malalignment). Exaggeration or flattening of these relatively normal cervical, thoracic, and lumbar curves is often seen in chronic spine and soft tissue injury conditions.

Standing Assessment

- Head position
- Shoulder position
- Cervical–thoracic–lumbar scoliosis
- Cervical–thoracic–lumbar (kyphosis/lordosis)
- Iliac crest (pelvis) alignment
- Hip/ knee position (flexed, externally/internally rotated)

It is also important to evaluate the patient in his or her normal sitting position. Poor sitting posture places excess strain on multiple structures, including the lumbar discs, cervical discs, and the low back and cervical musculature. Postural training, worksite evaluations, lumbar rolls, core strengthening, and stretching of tight musculature all can help to improve poor sitting posture.

Cervical and Lumbar Range of Motion

Cervical and lumbar range of motion (ROM) can be tested first actively (by the patient) and passively (by the clinician). Active range of motion, active assistive range of motion, and passive range of motion can be assessed for each joint. The examiner should note general hypermobility or hypomobility, side-to-side differences in range of motion, and which movements result in pain. Cervical testing includes cervical rotation (right/left), cervical flexion and extension, and cervical lateral bending on both sides. Lower extremity testing includes hip flexion/extension, hip adduction/abduction, hip internal/external rotation, knee flexion/extension, and foot dorsiflexion/plantar flexion.

Motor Strength

The clinician should also note any discomfort or pain reported by the patient during testing. Proper motor testing may be limited by multiple patient factors such as increased pain, affective distress, malingering (i.e., conscious feigning of symptoms).

Motor strength or power testing usually is localized to one joint. Strength testing is graded from 0 to 5 (full power), according to the Oxford Scale.

Motor Strength Testing

5 = Normal, full ROM vs. gravity, max resistance
4 = Good, full ROM vs. gravity, moderate resistance
3 = Fair, full ROM vs. gravity, no resistance
2 = Poor, full ROM, gravity eliminated
1 = Trace
0 = No activity

Strength testing may be limited by a patient's reports of pain and/or poor tolerance. Fatigue of muscles and relative weakness may also present with shaking of the limb during testing. Testing should progress in a structured manner from more proximal to distal muscle groups. Usually more than one muscle contributes to an isolated movement; single muscles are difficult to test. Focus on group movement and isolated movements. Commonly tested muscle groups include hip flexors (L2-L3), knee extension (L3-L4), knee flexors (L5-S1), ankle dorsiflexors (L4-L5), great toe extension (L5), and plantarflexors (S1-S2) (See Figures 4.1–4.5). Focal weakness may be consistent with nerve root or peripheral nerve compromise.

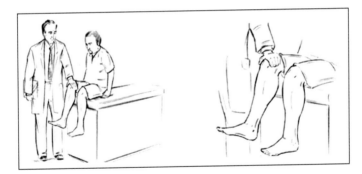

Figure 4.1 Testing hip flexion strength. *Source:* Permission to use storyboards was granted by Ortho-McNeil Janssen Scientific Affairs, LLC.

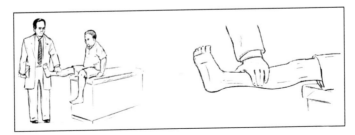

Figure 4.2 Testing knee extension strength. *Source:* Permission to use storyboards was granted by Ortho-McNeil Janssen Scientific Affairs, LLC.

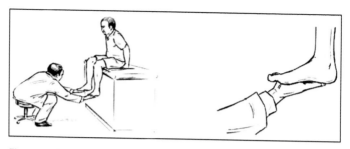

Figure 4.3 Testing ankle plantar flexion strength. *Source:* Permission to use storyboards was granted by Ortho-McNeil Janssen Scientific Affairs, LLC.

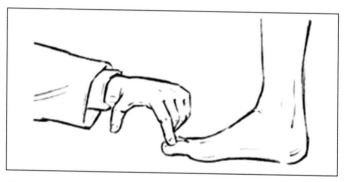

Figure 4.4 Testing great toe dorsiflexion. *Source:* Permission to use storyboards was granted by Ortho-McNeil Janssen Scientific Affairs, LLC.

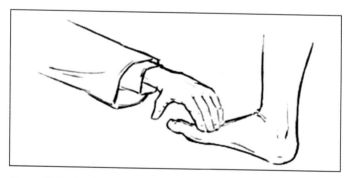

Figure 4.5 Testing ankle dorsiflexion. *Source:* Permission to use storyboards was granted by Ortho-McNeil Janssen Scientific Affairs, LLC.

Cervical and lumbar exam should include the following muscle groups:

Upper Limb Muscle Testing

C5, 6: Biceps
C6, 7: Wrist extensors
C7, 8: Triceps
C8, T1: Finger flexors
T1: Hand intrinsics

Lower Limb Muscle Testing

L1, 2, 3: Iliopsoas, quadriceps, hip adductors
L2, 3, 4: Quadriceps, ilopsoas, hip adductors
L3, 4, 5: Anterior tibialis, quadriceps, hamstrings
L4, 5: Extensor hallucis longus, gluteus maximus
S1: Gastrocnemius-soleus, peroneous longus, gluteus maximus

Sensation Testing

Sensation testing involves dull touch (fingertip), pin-prick (paper clip), and proprioception. Testing for the cervical dermatomes (C5–C8) and lumbar dermatones (L2-L5 and S1) is done by touching the skin in each sensory level. Clinicians should familiarize themselves with standard sensory and motor testing tools and diagrams, such as the standard neurological classification system published by the American Spinal Injury Association. Each sensory level is graded as reduced, normal, or increased.

Cervical Spine/Upper Extremity Sensation Testing

C5: Lateral side of antecubital fossa
C6: Thumb
C7: Middle finger
C8: Little finger
T1: Ulnar side of the antecubital fossa

Lower Extremity Sensation Testing

L2: Mid anterior thigh
L3: Medial femoral condyle
L4: Medial heel
L5: Dorsum of foot
S1: Lateral heel
S2: Popliteal fossa

Muscle Stretch Reflexes

Muscle stretch reflexes (deep tendon reflexes) are an important part of the spine-related exam. Loss of muscle reflex could be consistent with significant nerve root comprise or compression. Exaggerated reflex responses may be consistent with low motor neuron compromise (i.e., brain lesion, spinal cord mass, spinal cord compression).

The Queen Square hammer is preferred to the shorter "Taylor" or tomahawk hammer (Fig. 4.6).

It is important that the patient is relaxed and sitting comfortably. Each reflex is graded as absent/reduced, normal, or increased, as compared with the uninvolved extremity.

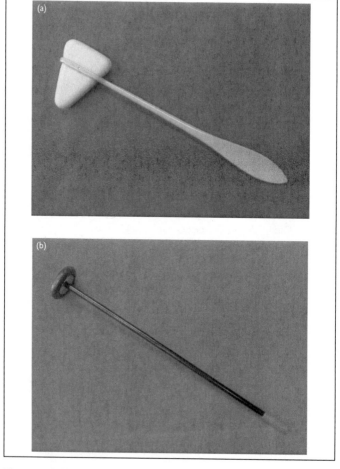

Figure 4.6 Reflex hammers. (a) Taylor or Tomahawk. (b) Queen Square.

Muscle Stretch Reflex Grading

4 + = hyperactive with clonus
3 + = more brisk
2 + = normal response
1 + = decreased with facilitation
0 = no response

Muscle stretch reflexes of the upper extremity involve the following muscles: biceps (C5–C6), brachioradialis (C5–C6), and triceps (C7).

Upper Limb Muscle Stretch Reflexes

Biceps: C5
Brachioradialis: C6
Triceps: C7

For the lower extremity, muscle stretch reflexes involve the following muscles: patella (L2, L3, L4), medial hamstring (L5, S1), and Achilles (S1, S2).

Lower Limb Muscle Stretch Reflexes

Patella: L4
Medial hamstring: L5
Achilles: S1

For the patellar muscle stretch reflex, have the patient sit with knee flexed. Strike the patellar tendon just below the patella. Observe the contraction of the quadriceps and extension of the knee. This test primarily evaluates the functionality of the L4 nerve root (See Figure 4.7).

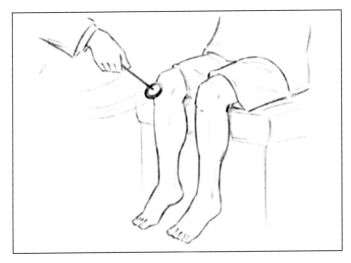

Figure 4.7 Testing patellar reflex. *Source:* Permission to use storyboards was granted by Ortho-McNeil Janssen Scientific Affairs, LLC.

Medial hamstring testing is also important, yet commonly ignored in the screening lumbar spine exam. The medial hamstrings (semitendinosus and semimembranous muscles) attach in the medial popliteal fossa, 1–2 cm above the tibial femoral joint line. Medial hamstring reflex is primarily innervated by the L5 and some S1 nerve root, via the tibial branch of the sciatic nerve. The medial hamstring reflex may be decreased or absent in patients with L5 disc herniations. It can be tested easily with the patient seated but also supine with the leg slightly flexed at the knee and externally rotated, or prone, with the knee flexed 90 degrees. The examiner should place fingers (usually index, long, and ring finger) in a cupped-like manner, grasping the insertion of the medial hamstrings at their insertion proximal to the knee. With the reflex hammer, strike the cupped fingers while supporting or pressing against the hamstrings where they insert distally at the knee.

For the Achilles muscle stretch reflex, dorsiflex the foot at the ankle slightly. Test for reflexes at both ankles (See Figure 4.8). Take note of bilateral or unilateral absence or inequality of the force of the responses from side to side. If the response is absent on one side or is weaker on one side, it may indicate compression of the S1 nerve root on that side. Absent reflexes on both sides may be normal for that patient but might indicate bilateral nerve root compression or a polyneuropathy. Also observe for a rhythmic or "beating" movement of the foot (clonus) (See Figure 4.9). The presence of clonus may be indicative of conditions affecting the spinal cord and indicates need for further neurologic evaluation.

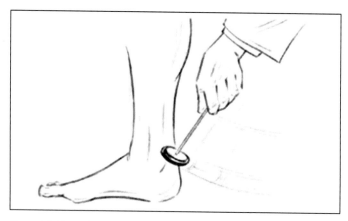

Figure 4.8 Testing Achilles reflex. *Source:* Permission to use storyboards was granted by Ortho-McNeil Janssen Scientific Affairs, LLC.

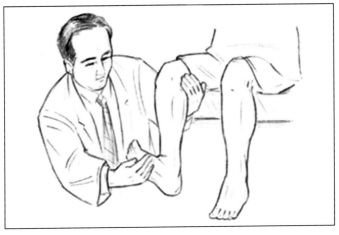

Figure 4.9 Testing ankle clonus. *Source:* Permission to use storyboards was granted by Ortho-McNeil Janssen Scientific Affairs, LLC.

Other Reflexes

Cervical myelopathy may result from pathologic compression of the spinal cord, and if significant enough, produce symptoms in the upper and lower limb. Decreased vibratory sense and proprioception distal to the lesion may be early signs. Other signs of myleopathy include hyperreflexia, Hoffman sign, ankle clonus, Babinski sign, and Oppenheim test.

For testing Babinski sign, run the end of a reflex hammer or an object with a blunted point up the lateral border of the foot and across the metatarsal pads to the medial side of the foot (See Figure 4.10). Note the movement of the toes. Plantar flexion of the toes is normal, or a negative Babinski sign, whereas extension of the big toe and fanning of other toes indicates a positive Babinski sign. A positive Babinski sign may be indicative of a condition that has affected the central nervous system, including the brain or spinal cord, and indicates need for further neurologic evaluation.

Provocative Testing of the Upper Extremities

Dural Tension: Radiculopathy, Peripheral Nerve Pathology

Radiculopathy may be due to compression of a single cervical or lumbar root secondary to a disk herniation, producing a single level deficit with normal motor and sensory testing above and below the affected nerve root level.

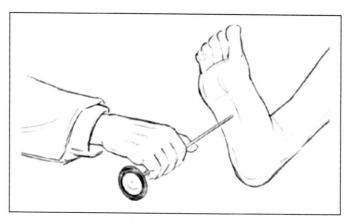

Figure 4.10 Testing Babinski reflex. *Source:* Permission to use storyboards was granted by Ortho-McNeil Janssen Scientific Affairs, LLC.

Physical findings may include an asymmetric and/or reduced muscle stretch reflex, motor weakness, atrophy of muscle, sensory impairment (decreased light touch or pin sensation), and cervical neural tension.

A number of provocative tests for cervical radiculopathy may be used, including Spurling Test, the Shoulder Abduction Test, and Upper Limb Tension Testing.

Spurling Test: Patient is seated, the neck is passively side-bent toward the symptomatic side, and overpressure is applied to the patient's head. Note reproduction of patient's symptoms (radiation of pain down upper extremity).

Shoulder Abduction Test: The patient is seated and asked to place the hand of the symptomatic extremity on the head. A positive test occurs when symptoms are reduced or eliminated in the distal limb.

Neck Distraction Test: The patient is supine while the examiner grasps under the chin and occiput, flexes the patient's neck to position of comfort, and gradually applies a superiorly directed distraction force up to 14 kg. A positive test occurs with reduction or elimination of symptoms.

Upper Limb Tension Test: Patient is supine while the examiner sequentially introduces (1) scapular depression, (2) shoulder abduction, (3) forearm supination, wrist and finger extension, (4) shoulder lateral rotation, (5) elbow extension, and (6) contralateral then ipsilateral cervical side-bending.

Peripheral Nerve Screen: Upper Extremity

It may be prudent at this point in the exam to consider screening median and ulnar neuropathy, while checking dural tension in the upper extremities. The etiology of these types of neuropathy is the result of compression of the peripheral nerve itself, causing distal symptoms of tingling, pain (paresthesias), numbness, and if prolonged and severe enough, weakness.

Median Nerve Testing

The median nerve innervates mainly muscles in the distal arm, and it is responsible for pronation and flexion of the forearm, flexion and abduction of the wrist, flexion of the MCP and PIP joints, and in particular, flexion, opposition, and abduction of the thumb. The most common cause of median neuropathy is compression of the median nerve while in the carpal tunnel (carpal tunnel syndrome).

Phalen Test: Patient places both hands in a maximally flexed position for about one minute. The test is positive when symptoms are reproduced in the first, second, third, and the radial half of the fourth digit.

Compression Test: Patient's arm is supinated and the examiner provides pressure to the carpal tunnel while grasping the wrist with both hands and thumbs overlapped. The test is positive when symptoms are reproduced in the first, second, third, and the radial half of the fourth digit.

Tinel Test: The examiner taps the volar wrist (carpal tunnel) with a reflex hammer. The test is positive when symptoms are reproduced in the first, second, third, and the radial half of the fourth digit.

Ulnar Nerve Testing

The ulnar nerve also innervates muscles of the forearm, and in particular is responsible for finger adduction of all fingers, abduction of all fingers except thumb, flexion of the fourth and fifth digits, wrist flexion, and adduction. The ulnar nerve travels along the ulnar groove found by the medial epicondyle of the elbow proximally (cubital canal) and distally over the hamate bone in Guyon canal. The most common cause of ulnar neuropathy is compression in these two areas.

Tinel Test: Similar to the median nerve testing, except the examiner taps the medial elbow with a reflex hammer. The test is positive when symptoms are reproduced in the fifth and ulnar half of the fourth digit.

Provocative Testing of the Lower Extremities/ Lumbosacral Spine

A number of provocative tests for checking dural tension in the form of lumbar radiculopathy that may be used include Straight Leg Raise, Slump Sit Test, and Femoral Nerve Stretch. Other provocative maneuvers to test for sacroiliac joint dysfunction and pain include sacroiliac joint (SIJ) border tenderness testing, Patrick test, Gaenslen test, and Compression testing.

Dural Tension: Lower Extremity/Lumbosacral Spine

Straight Leg Raise: Pain occurs in the ipsilateral leg as the leg is elevated between 30 and 60 degrees when patient is supine on the exam table. If pain increases by flexing the ankle while the leg is raised, this is another indicator of nerve root involvement. The straight leg raise test is a sensitive but not a very specific indicator of nerve root compression. (See Fig. 4.11.)

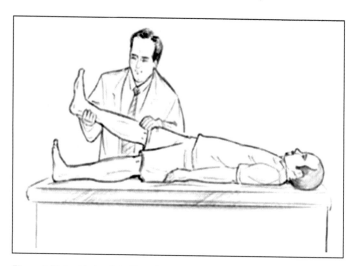

Figure 4.11 Straight Leg Raise Test. *Source:* Permission to use storyboards was granted by Ortho-McNeil Janssen Scientific Affairs, LLC.

Cross Straight Leg Raise Test: Similar to the straight leg raise test, but it is considered positive when pain radiates into the contralateral leg. The cross straight leg raise is more specific but less sensitive for the presence of lumbosacral nerve root compression. Note the patient's responses as to when he or she feels pain and whether with only one leg versus the other or both. Pain and discomfort during this test may indicate compression of the lower nerve roots, including L4, L5, and S1. (See Fig. 4.12.)

Slump Sit Test: Patient sits at edge of exam table with hands clasped behind back and head flexed down to chest. The examiner should first test the unaffected side, then the affected side, by raising the leg with knee extended. The test is positive if radiation of pain is reproduced and if pain is improved when head is raised from flexed position.

Femoral Nerve Stretch: Patient is in prone position on exam table, while the examiner maximally flexes the knee on each side. This stresses the femoral nerve. The test is positive when pain is produced in the lumbar area, buttock, or posterior thigh.

Sacroiliac Joint Dysfunction

The sacroiliac joints (SIJ) help transmit weight from the spine to the lower extremities while acting as a shock absorber. Over time and with aging, pathology can develop in these joints, compromising their function and leading to pain and dysfunction.

SIJ Border Tenderness: Pain from the sacroiliac joint is commonly referred to a small area (approximately 3 x 10 cm) inferior and medial to the ipsilateral posterior superior iliac spine and may be easily predicted by the patient pointing with one finger to this area.[1,2]

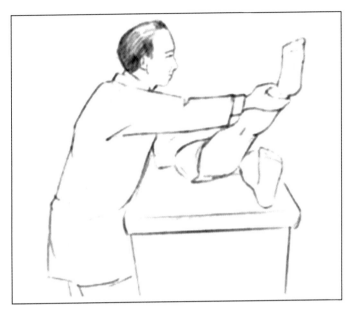

Figure 4.12 Cross Straight Leg Raise Test. *Source:* Permission to use storyboards was granted by Ortho-McNeil Janssen Scientific Affairs, LLC.

Patrick Test: Sometimes known as the FABERE test, it involves testing the patient in the supine position with the following maneuvers performed on the lower extremities: Flexion, Abduction, External Rotation, and Extension. Pain may be elicited on the ipsilateral leg on which maneuver is performed. A test is positive only when it produces concordant pain response. The patient endorses pain reproduction in the buttock and/or along the sacroiliac joint region, not the lumbar spine.

Gaenslen Test: Patient is in the supine position, flexes ipsilateral hip and knee (patient aids by grasping firmly his or her own leg), bringing the lumbar spine in contact with the examination table. Patient is then shifted laterally to edge of table so as to hyperextend the contralateral leg below the level of the table. The test is positive when pain is localized in the sacroiliac joint area (buttock or referred pain regions) on the side of the extended leg.

Compression Testing: Also sometimes referred to as midline sacral thrust. The patient lies laterally on one side and the examiner exerts medial force on the anterior superior iliac spine (ASIS). The test is positive if pain is elicited in SIJ or gluteal region.

Myofascial or Soft Tissue Assessment

Passive testing also affords the opportunity to examine related myofascial pain generators in the related cervical and lumbar paraspinal areas. Myofascial pain assessment is important and highly prevalent with neck and low back pain; it can be a primary or secondary cause of dysfunction and pain, many times due to direct or indirect trauma, exposure to cumulative activity, postural dysfunction, and deconditioning.[3]

Trigger points (TPs) are characterized by tender, firm nodules (3–6 mm in size) found on palpatory exam.[4] Original diagnostic criteria for the diagnosis of TPs include tenderness within taut bands of muscle, characteristic and predictable patterns of referred pain within the taut band, and limited painful range of motion.

Trigger points can be classified as "active" (symptomatic) or "latent" (asymptomatic). Active points usually coincide with the patient's individual complaints, as compared to "latent" points, which usually are found on exam by the practitioner. Light palpation along the cervical paraspinals parallel to the orientation of the muscle fibers may help to localize painful areas and focal myofascial trigger points. Classic referral patterns from cervical and lumbar areas can be assessed and many times may be confused with referral patterns of radiculopathy. With regard to cervical and lumbar pain, the TPs pattern of referral from the cervical and lumbar spine may refer pain to the head and upper extremity (cervical) and the lower leg (lumbar).

Myofascial Trigger Pain Referral Patterns

Head, Trunk, and Upper Extremities

Trapezius
Levator scapulae
Posterior cervical area
Sternal area
Serratus anterior
Scalenes
Supraspinatus
Infraspinatus
Pectoralis

Lumbar and Lower Extremities

Longissimus dorsi
Gluteus maximus
Gluteus minimus
Adductor longus
Biceps femoris
Tibialis anterior

Balance and Proprioception

Balance can be assessed via Romberg Testing, which involves having the patient standing with the feet shoulder-width apart, eyes closed. The examiner taps the patient on the shoulder from unexpected directions; normal testing will show that patient is able to maintain his or her balance.

Proprioceptive testing can be performed for the upper and lower extremities. The examiner holds the thumb or the great toe at the lateral bony joint line, without touching any other digits. The examiner first demonstrates movement, for example, up or down. Then the patient is asked to close his or her eyes and asked to report the direction of movement that the examiner exerts.

Gait should also be assessed in order to better assess balance and proprioceptive conditions (cerebellar lesions, posterior column injury, or pathology). Cervical myelopathic compression may also lead to lower extremity dysfunction and gait abnormalities. Gait can be thought of as a cycle of each foot with two phases: stance and swing. The skills required for competent gait analysis can take years of experience to acquire, and accordingly, the following is meant as a basic overview to help identify major and/or common pathology.

Antalgic Gait: This is a gait in which a patient appears to favor one leg over the other due to pain.

Trendelenburg Gait: This type of gait appears with weakness of the gluteus medius muscle. It can be tested by having the patient stand on one leg while raising the other. Normal strength of the gluteus medius on the stance leg will show no alteration of the pelvis. Weakness of the gluteus medius on the stance leg will result in inability to exert full abduction on the hip and cause the pelvis to dip down on the contralateral side.

Circumduction: Weak hip flexor muscles are unable to lift the knee high enough to clear the foot from the floor. The compensatory movement is circumduction, in which the patient performs a lateral circular movement of the lower extremity (abduction, external rotation, adduction, and internal rotation).

Hip Hiking: During the swing phase, the patient will attempt to raise the hip up on the side that has increased functional leg length due to hip weakness and/or extensor spasticity of the lower leg.

Foot Slap: Weak muscles responsible for dorsiflexion of the foot will cause the patient to slap his or her forefoot down as the heel strikes. It can also be accompanied by steppage gait, in which there is excessive hip and knee flexion during stance phase.

Toe Drag: Weak dorsiflexor muscles of the foot can also cause toe drag, which does not allow the forefoot and toes to fully clear the floor during swing phase.

Pain Behavior

Although often overlooked or recorded in routine exams, patient pain behaviors or "illness behavior" are important parts of the comprehensive chronic pain assessment. As proposed originally by Fordyce, "pain behaviors" are based on operant contingency models of reinforcement and act as a means for the patient to communicate to the environment that he or she is experiencing pain or distress.[5] Pain behaviors, which can be thought of as behavioral manifestations of pain (i.e., grimacing, complaining, inactivity) may be reinforced in both a positive and negative manner. For example, by obtaining attention from family members and being excused from undesirable obligations such as work or pain-provoking activities, the patient may gain in a "positive" way. In a similar scenario, the patient grimacing in pain may receive negative reinforcement from family members, who may make the patient feel guilty for having a pain problem and being unable to work and provide for the family. These reinforcement contingencies, primarily positive ones, many times remain long after the precipitation injury (i.e., tissue trauma) has resolved.

Other pain behaviors include guarding, bracing, rubbing the painful area, facial grimacing and sighing,[6] distortion of ambulation or posture, and negative affect.[7]

Pain behavior may also manifest with the use of devices, including walking devices (canes, crutches) and equipment (braces, splints, cold or heat packs).

Pain Behavior: Common Signs

- Grimacing
- Guarding
- Screaming or verbalizing pain with movement
- Antalgic gait pattern
- Equipment
- Modality devices (cold and ice packs, TENS units)

Pain behaviors have been found to correlate with self-report measures of pain intensity, pain disability, and self-efficacy,[8] and they may serve as targets for cognitive and behavioral treatment and in turn can be "unlearned."

Waddell and Main described illness behavior as "what people say and do to express and communicate they are ill."[9] Waddell classically described seven nonanatomic signs or behavioral symptoms in patients with low back pain, which are known as the Waddell signs. These seven signs were standardized into five general categories: tenderness, simulation, distraction, regional complaints, and overreaction. In their initial study, which included a cohort of low back pain patients, patients displaying at least three signs were more likely to have evidence of psychosocial distress.[10]

Although controversial, there is no consistent evidence that Waddell signs are associated with malingering, the intentional production of false or grossly exaggerated physical or psychological symptoms, or secondary gain, defined as interpersonal advantages one obtains as the result of injury or disease.[11] Fishbain et al. demonstrated that Waddell signs were not associated with physician perception of effort exaggeration and found evidence that Waddell signs decreased with comprehensive pain treatment.[12]

Summary

Physical exam for neck and lumbar or lower extremity pain incorporates a range of neurologic, musculoskeletal, and myofascial tests and assessments. A thorough examination is an extension of a focused and comprehensive history.

These tests will help rule in or rule out specific pain generators and help the clinician to better understand more complex findings. For example, multiple abnormalities may be found, including, abnormal postures, chronic muscle imbalances or weakness, myofascial and compensatory soft tissue, and gait abnormalities. Provocative testing may include tests to recreate facet joint, sacroiliac joint, and radiculopathy, or peripheral nerve dysfunction.

Any exam relies on a foundation of accurate basic physical examination, including joint range of motion, sensory and muscle stretch reflex testing, motor strength, and balance. With any patient, whether the complaint is acute or chronic, related pain behavior should also be assessed and documented. Underlying pain behavior may help identify affective distress (depression, anxiety) and clue the clinician to other operant or psychosocial factors.

References

1 Fortin JD, Dwyer AP, West S, Pier J. Sacroiliac joint: pain referral maps upon applying a new injection/ arthrography technique. I: asymptomatic volunteers. *Spine.* 1994;19:1475–1482.

2 .Fortin JD, Falco FJ. The Fortin finger test: an indicator of sacroiliac pain. *Am J Orthop.* 1997;26:477–480.

3 Wheeler AH, Aaron GW. Muscle pain due to injury. *Curr Pain Headache Rep.* 2001;5:441–446.

4 Simons DG, Travell JG, Simons LS. *Travell and Simons' Myofascial Pain Dysfunction: The Trigger Point Manual.* 2nd ed. Baltimore, Md: Williams & Wilkins; 1999.

5 Fordyce WE. *Behavioral Methods for Chronic Pain and Illness.* St. Louis, Mo: Mosby; 1976.

6 Keefe FJ, Block AR, Williams RB Jr, Surwit RS. Behavioral treatment of chronic low back pain: clinical outcome and individual differences in pain relief. *Pain.* 1981;11(2):221–231.

7 Turk DC, Wack JT, Kerns RD. An empirical examination of the "pain-behavior" construct. *J Behav Med.* 1985;8(2):119–130.

8 McCahon S, Strong J, Sharry R, Cramond T. Self-report and pain behavior among patients with chronic pain. *Clin J Pain.* 2005;21(3):223–231.

9 Main CJ, Waddell G. Behavioral responses to examination. A reappraisal of the interpretation of "nonorganic signs". *Spine.* 1998;23(21):2367–2371.

10 Main CJ, Waddell G. Behavioral responses to examination. A reappraisal of the interpretation of "nonorganic signs". *Spine.* 1998;23(21):2367–2371.

11 Fishbain DA, Rosomoff HL, Cutler RB, et al. Secondary gain concept: a review of the scientific evidence. *Clin J Pain.* 1995;11:6–21.

12 Fishbain DA, Cutler RB, Rosomoff HL, Rosomoff RS. Is there a relationship between nonorganic physical findings (Waddell Signs) and secondary gain/malingering? *Clin J Pain.* 2004;20(6):399–408.

Chapter 5

Difficult-to-Treat Pain Syndromes

Yvonne D'Arcy

Some conditions with chronic persistent pain are more difficult to manage than pain from an acute injury. These patients are those that have high pain ratings consistently no matter how medications or interventions are manipulated. Finding the right combination of treatment options can provide the best possible outcome with increased satisfaction for both patients and providers.

Fibromyalgia Syndrome

There has been much written and discussed about the cause of fibromyalgia and how to diagnose and treat the condition. Fibromyalgia syndrome (FMS) has long been considered a diagnosis of exclusion and because of that aspect, it can take up to 5 years for a patient with fibromyalgia to obtain the diagnosis. However, for the fibromyalgia patient, the onset of a chronic debilitating condition that limits activity, interferes with sleep, and provides constant pain is a life-changing event. The fact that mood disturbances and personality disorders can accompany pain complaints with fibromyalgia further complicates the clinical presentation of the patient. To add further confusion, patients may also have comorbidities such as lupus, osteoarthritis, rheumatoid arthritis, or Sjogren syndrome.[1]

There are some commonalities among patients who have fibromyalgia.[2,3,4] Patients can complain of the following:

- Painful tender points at multiple sites on the body
- Sleep disturbance
- Fatigue
- Mood disturbances

Less commonly, patients can complain of the following:

- Cognitive loss
- Irritable bowel or bladder
- Restless legs
- Temporomandibular joint pain
- Anxiety, depression, or panic attacks

For patients who have fibromyalgia, these complaints and pain can severely limit normal everyday living. FMS is more common in women than in men. Overall, it occurs in about 2%–5% of the U.S. population, 3.5%–7% of women and only 0.5%–2% of men.[2] There is no specific trigger that has been implicated in the development of fibromyalgia, but chronic stress, genetic susceptibility, or early childhood trauma have all been considered as potential contributors to the development of FMS.

What we do know is that fibromyalgia patients have 2–5 times the amount of substance P, a pain facilitating substance, in their cerebrospinal fluid.[3] Studies that are more recent have focused on the activation of the central nervous system with magnetic resonance imaging (MRI) scans during pain stimulation, leading to the premise that fibromyalgia is really a centrally mediated pain syndrome accounting for the diverse location of the painful tender points.[5] No matter what the cause of the syndrome, fibromyalgia remains difficult to diagnose and treat.

Assessment

The diagnosis of FMS is difficult to make because not all FMS patients present the same. In 1990, The American College of Rheumatology (ACR) developed criteria that are used to diagnose FMS. These criteria are as follows:

- Widespread bilateral pain above and below the waist of at least 3 months duration
- Excessive tenderness on applying pressure to 11 of 18 muscle-tendon sites (tender points; see Fig. 5.1)

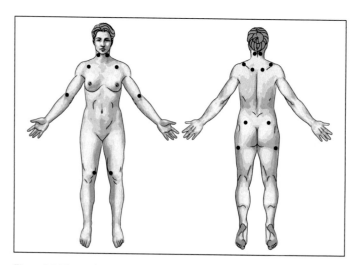

Figure 5.1 Fibromyalgia tender points.

There is also a Manual Tender Point Survey that can be useful for standardizing the assessment and diagnosis procedures.[3] This tool gives specific instructions on how to perform a tender point assessment and provides the specific locations for testing. Using this tool for the initial diagnosis will provide a baseline for comparison with later assessment. Newer criteria from the ACR use the tender point survey in conjunction with a patient questionnaire detailing symptom severity in order to give greater clarity to the diagnostic criteria for fibromyalgia.[6]

Another assessment tool that is helpful in determining the effects of fibromyalgia on the patient's quality of life and functionality is the Fibromyalgia Impact Questionnaire (FIQ). The FIQ is a short 10-item self-administered assessment tool that assesses the patient's status in physical functioning, work status, depression, anxiety, sleep, pain, stiffness, fatigue, and well-being. It is reliable and valid and can be very useful in comparing assessments to track progress.[3]

Treating Fibromyalgia Syndrome

There are a variety of treatment approaches to FMS, including medications and other types of integrative medicine options. After the diagnosis has been made and the symptoms persist or worsen, the APS Fibromyalgia Guidelines (2005) recommend sleep hygiene, referrals to community exercise programs, relaxation techniques, patient education, and cognitive-behavioral therapy.

Treatments with Modest to Strong Evidence for Efficacy
Medications

- Dual reuptake inhibitors (SNRIs), such as duloxetine 60 mg per day and milnacipran 50 mg twice per day (FDA approved for FMS)
- Pregabalin 75 mg b.i.d. (FDA approved for FMS)
- Amitriptyline 20–50 mg
- Cyclobenzaprine 10–30 mg
- Tramadol 200–300 mg
- Selective serotonin reuptake inhibitors (SSRIs), fluoxetine 60 mg day (Higher doses of older serotonin drugs appear to work in fibromyalgia because at higher doses they seem to block the reuptake of norepinephrine as well as serotonin.)

Other Modalities

- Cognitive-behavioral therapies
- Cardiovascular exercise
- Patient education
- Biofeedback
- Acupuncture
- Hypnotherapy
- Multidisciplinary treatment programs

Treatments with No Evidence for Efficacy

- Opioids
- Corticosteroids

- Melatonin
- Calcitonin
- Guaifenesin
- DHEA
- Nonsteroidal anti-inflammatory drugs (NSAIDs)
- Benzodiazipines
- Trigger point injections
- Flexibility exercise
- Nutritional, herbs, other complementary and alternative medicine therapy (APS, 2005)

For many years fibromyalgia patients were told that their complaints were "all in your head." With today's ability to see the actual pain being produced on MRI scans, the root of the pain can be seen and accepted. The FMS patient no longer must learn to put up with the pain and regard the illness as imaginary. There are new methods for diagnosis and treatment that can make the symptoms of the condition tolerable and allow the patient to have a more productive and functional life despite FMS.

Myofascial Pain Syndromes

Myofascial pain syndromes (MPS) are common pain complaints. The conditions have been called by a variety of names such as fibrositis or musculoskeletal pain disorders.[7] The complaint has been associated with low back pain, neck and shoulder pain, arthritis, tension headaches, and the general term *primary myalgia*.[8]

The defining characteristic of myofascial pain, whether it is acute, chronic, regional, or widespread, is that it is associated with pain or tenderness localized to a linear or nodular hardening in a muscle that is called a myofascial trigger point.[6] There was consideration in earlier years that myofascial pain and fibromyalgia were similar if not the same. Current thinking is that FMS is part of a group of diseases that are characterized by systemic symptoms with muscle pain possibly representing a type of central sensitization, while MPS is primarily a muscle pain disorder.[5]

MPS is defined by the presence of painful trigger points in a taut band of muscle that can produce referred pain with palpation. As time progresses, hypersensitivity or allodynia can develop at the site of the inflammatory process.[6] Three essential characteristics are considered necessary for a diagnosis of MPS:

- Regional pain
- Presence of trigger points
- Normal findings on neurological examination

Other findings that are considered to be consistent with diagnosing MPS by 80% of practitioners who were surveyed on the topic included the following[5]:

- Muscular tender points
- Taut bands

- Muscle ropiness or muscle nodules
- Dull, achy, or deep pain
- Decreased range of motion
- Pain that is exacerbated by stress

MPS can be caused by a variety of conditions such as whiplash, repetitive muscle overload, postural imbalance, or injured or inflamed muscles.[6] The resultant muscle spasm, muscle tightening, and pain can start as an acute condition and progress to more chronic and debilitating conditions such as frozen shoulder, piriformis syndrome, interscalene compartment syndrome, thoracic outlet syndrome, chronic headaches, or temporomandibular joint syndrome.[6] Referrals for physical therapy and occupational therapy are the first step in developing a treatment plan for patients with MPS.

Treating the Pain of Myofascial Pain Syndromes

Medication Management[5,6]

Because of the diverse nature of MPS there are a variety of medications that are effective for treating pain:

- NSAIDs such as ketoprofen or celecoxib
- Steroid taper in the early stage
- Muscle relaxants
- Tricyclic antidepressants and venlafaxine
- Anticonvulsants
- Antispasticity drugs such as tizanidine
- Opioids analgesics
- Botulinum toxin

Physical Modalities

- Trigger point injections, compression, stretch
- Therapeutic spray and stretch
- Myofascial release
- Muscle reeducation
- Dry needling or injection
- Massage
- Ultrasound
- Acupuncture
- Electrical stimulation

Although the pain of MPS is significant and causes a loss of functionality and quality of life there is still no definitive answer to the best treatment or options. The most commonly tried approach is trigger point injection in the early stages. The goal of treatment is maintenance of physical strength and mobility; collaboration with physical therapy is necessary to achieve the best outcomes for the patient.

Pain with Whiplash or Whiplash Associated Disorders

Whiplash injuries can occur as a result of a rear-end collision or side collision from a motor vehicle accident. It is defined as "a process of hyperextension and hyperflexion of the cervical musculature."[9] The other element that has been cited as defining whiplash is an acceleration-deceleration mechanism of energy transfer to the neck. It may result from rear-end or side-impact motor vehicle collisions, but it can also occur while driving or other mishaps. The impact may result in bony or soft tissue injuries (whiplash-injury), which in turn may lead to a variety of clinical manifestations called whiplash-associated disorders (WAD).[10]

Overall, the quick forward and backward motion of the neck can result in a painful injury that can limit motion and activity and progress to a chronic condition that is more difficult to treat.

Whiplash and WAD are very common disorders. The incidence has been estimated to be from one case per 1000 inhabitants in Western societies, to 70 per 100,000 in Quebec, to 106 per 100,000 in Australia.[7,8] Whiplash injuries usually resolve in a short period of time. It is estimated that approximately 20% to 40% of the injuries progress to some form of chronic pain complaint when the data include international statistics.

Characteristics of pain reported by patients with whiplash and WAD include the following:

- Present at rest and with cervical rotation, flexion, and extension
- Interference with personal activities
- Difficulty with lifting
- Dizziness and interference with concentration
- Headaches
- Sleep disturbances
- Some pain may radiate down one or both arms; shoulder pain
- Visual or auditory symptoms
- Dysphagia
- Paresthesias

Patients with WAD are classified by the severity of the signs and symptoms of the injury:

Grade 0:	No complaints or physical signs
Grade 1:	Neck complaints (pain, tenderness, and stiffness) but no physical signs
Grade 2:	Neck complaints and musculoskeletal signs (decreased range of motion or muscle weakness)
Grade 3 and 4:	Neck complaints and neurological signs, fractures or dislocation

In an effort to determine which patients might progress to a chronic condition, a Cochrane review has determined that high pain intensity ratings after injury is the most predictive factor for developing a chronic pain condition after whiplash injury.[11] Other factors that were weakly associated with predicting disability were as follows:

- Driving as an occupation
- High initial pain intensity
- Restricted neck movement
- Low muscle workload
- High number of complaints
- Previous psychological problems[11]

The findings also indicated that 82% of patients who were diagnosed with WAD were free of symptoms 2 years after the injury.[11]

Assessing Pain in Patients with Whiplash and Whiplash Associated Disorders

To assess patients with whiplash and WAD, a specialized assessment tool, the Neck Disability Index (NDI), has been developed. It is a reliable and valid tool that is designed to be viewed as a two-factor instrument; pain and interference with cognitive functioning, and functional disability.[9] The function and disability factor is associated with items in the NDI pertaining to personal care, lifting, concentration, work, driving, and recreation, while the pain intensity factor is focused on items that are related to headache, neck pain, reading, and sleeping.[9] Although more research is needed on the specific subscales of this instrument, it currently provides a method for assessing some of the major areas of WAD and a means to measure outcomes.

One very important aspect of whiplash injuries is the progression to a chronic condition that requires work disability. In a cohort study of patients with WAD, followed out to 12 months after the accident, age and concentration impairment were independent predictors of long-lasting work disability.[12] The author suggests that progress could be made in decreasing WAD-related disability if interventions were aimed more at restoring cognition rather than focusing solely on physical disability.

Treatment Options for Patients with Whiplash and Whiplash Associated Disorders

There are a variety of treatment options for patients with whiplash injuries encompassing a wide variety of choices. Most choices are focused on more conservative options, and research support has been limited by the variety of studies, which makes pooling data more difficult. Some of the more common conservative treatment options include the following[13,14]:

- Local heat and ice
- Neck collar immobilization (should not be overused)
- Ultrasound
- Traction
- Massage
- Exercises
- (Active) mobilization

- Ultrasound
- Multimodal rehabilitation

More aggressive treatment options for whiplash include interventional or surgical options. As with the conservative options, the research base is somewhat limited by the lack of high-quality studies, the results of which could be pooled to better predict outcomes. Some of the more common interventional and surgical treatment options include the following:

- Radiofrequency neurotomy
- Steroid injections
- Botulinum treatments
- Carpal tunnel decompression
- Cervical discectomy

The results of a large systematic review indicate that there is little evidence to recommend one therapy over another. This does not mean that the therapies are not effective, only that the research on the various therapies is not complete enough to make a recommendation. One of the biggest limitations of the research thus far is that many of the studies have been comparison studies of treatments with few having a follow-up to test for long-term efficacy. However, results from individual studies do indicate some advantages of one therapy over another.

Moderate Level of Evidence

- Acupuncture when tested against sham acupuncture[15]
- Mobilization[16]
- Intravenous methylprednisolone-reduced pain short term but not long term[17]
- Radio-frequency neurotomy for patients with pain >3 months[18]

Limited Evidence

- Chiropractic
- Muscle relaxants, analgesics, and nonsteroidal anti-inflammatory drugs (NSAIDs)

Not Effective

- Exercise alone
- Botulinum toxin injections give similar results as saline placebo
- Patient education, neck school, advice on stress coping skills[19]

For most patients with acute whiplash injury, maintaining mobility will help decrease pain and avoid a misuse syndrome. Using medications for pain relief is only for symptomatic treatments and to keep the patients active. Creating the idea that medication is a means to promoting wellness and activity, rather than a reliance on medication alone, is important.

Interventional modalities should be limited to patients who have had the pain for an extended period of time. For these patients it is important for them to work toward recovery or increased functionality rather than sinking into a helpless, hopeless state.

Summary

All of the pain conditions in this chapter can be debilitating and can impair quality of life for patients. They can also be very difficult for practitioners to treat since the end goal may be symptom management rather than cure. Using evidence-based options and national guideline recommendations will help provide the best outcome possible for difficult to treat pain syndromes.

References

1 Bennett RM. The rational management of fibromyalgia patients. *Rheum Dis Clin North Am.* 2002;28(2):1-16.

2 Goldenburg DL, Burkhardt C, Crofford L. Management of fibromyalgia syndrome. *J Am Med Soc.* 2004;292(12):2388-2394.

3 American Pain Society. *Fibromyalgia Pain Guidelines.* Glenview, Ill: The Society; 2005.

4 D'Arcy Y, McCarberg B. New fibromyalgia pain management recommendations. *The Nurse Practitioner Journal* 2005;Nov/Dec:31-40.

5 Mease P, Berney S, Arnold L, et al. Fibromyalgia diagnostic and treatment challenges: results from a recent summit of fibromyalgia experts. (Medscape # 701757) [Accessed September, 2010.]

6 Wolfe F, Clauw DJ, Fitzcharles MA, et al. The American College of Rheumatology preliminary diagnostic criteria for fibromyalgia and measurement of symptom severity. *Arthritis Care Res.* 2010;62(5):600-610.

7 Harden N. Muscle pain syndromes. *Phys Med Rehab.* 2007;86(1):S47-S58.

8 Gerwin R. Myofascial pain and fibromyalgia. In: Wallace MS, Staats P, eds. *Just the Facts: Pain Medicine.* New York, NY: McGraw Hill; 2005:204-209.

9 Neito R, Miro J, Huguet A. Disability in subacute whiplash patients: usefulness of the neck disability index. *Spine.* 2008;33(18):E630-E635.

10 Verhagen A, Scholten-Peeters G, Vanwijngaarden S. deBie R, Blerma-Zeinstra S. Conservative treatments for whiplash. *Cochrane Database Sys Rev.* 2007;2:CD003338.

11 Scholten-Peters G, Verhagen A, Bekkering G, et al. Prognostic factors of whiplash associated disorders: a systematic review of prospective cohort studies. *Pain.* 2003;104:303-322.

12 Buitenhius J, deJong P, Jaspers J, Groothoff J. Work disability after whiplash: a prospective cohort study. *Spine.* 2009;34(3):262-267.

13 Conlin A, Bhogal S, Sequeira K, Teasall R. Treatment of whiplash disorders-part I: noninvasive interventions. *Pain Res Manag.* 2009;10(1):21-32.

14 Conlin A, Bhogal S, Sequeira K, Teasall R. Treatment of whiplash disorders-part II: medical and surgical interventions. *Pain Res Manag.* 2005;10(1):33-40.

15 Trinh K, Graham N, Gross A, et al. Acupuncture for neck disorders. *Cochrane Database Sys Rev.* 2006;3:CD004870.

16 Rosenfeld M, Gunnarsson R, Borenstien P. Early intervention in whiplash-associated disorders. A comparison of two treatment protocols. *Spine.* 2000;15(25):1782-1787.

17 Peloso P, Michael J, Gross A, et al. Medicinal and injection therapies for mechanical neck disorders. *Cochrane Database Sys Rev.* 2007;3:CD000319.

18 Scherokman B, Gross A. Review: manual therapy in combination with other treatments may provide short-term relief in mechanical neck pain. *ACP Journal Club.* 2007;126:70.

19 Haines T, Gross A, Burnie S, Goldsmith C, Perry L. Patient education for neck pain with or without radiculopathy. *Cochrane Database Sys Rev.* 2009;1:CD005106.

Chapter 6

Disability Management in Primary Care: Practical Overview of Assessment and Services

Steven Stanos

Approximately 50 to 60 million people in the United States live with conditions that may be related to a disability.[1] Neck pain has a lifetime prevalence of 70% in the general population and up to 19% of the population may suffer from chronic neck pain at any given time.[2,3] Measuring the impact of neck pain is an ongoing challenge due to variability among patients with regard to pain intensity and related effects on physical and psychosocial functioning.[4,5]

A recent study of patients with chronic whiplash associated disorder found psychological factors, including fear avoidance beliefs and pain amplification, influenced self-ratings of perceived disability.[6] Besides physical and psychological factors, presence of a primary family member or spouse with a work-related spine disability was also found to be a risk factor for the development of disability.[7]

Low back pain remains the leading cause of disability in persons less than 45 years old.[8] Low back pain alone is estimated to cost up to $118 billion annually in the United States.[9] Although most acute low back pain episodes are assumed to be self-limiting in nature, recurrence within 1 year varies. Recurrence of acute low back pain after a period of compete resolution of symptoms varies considerably, but it may be greater at 1 year in patients with a previous history of low back pain.[10] Conservative estimates suggest up to 8% of patients may progress to chronic low back pain after a single low back pain episode.[11]

Pain Theory

Historically, conceptual models of pain and pain-related disability initially described pain as a purely sensory phenomenon. Gradually, these models evolved to include a more holistic mind-body approach, including Hippocrates and Galen's (c. 150 CE) description of the imbalance of bodily "humors" as a means of developing chronic pain and suffering.

55

A more biomedical model that concentrated on identifying and reversing, or eliminating pain, served as the focus of pain treatment during its early development in the 1950s. In 1965, Melzack and Wall proposed the gate control theory of pain, which proposed that pain experience was determined by physical, motivational, cognitive, and emotional factors, and transmission of nerve impulses could be modulated by a spinal gating mechanism at the level of the dorsal horn.[12] Melzack furthered this more dynamic role of pain networks with the "neuromatrix" model, championing the brain and central nervous system to be individually affected by both genetic and environmental stimuli.[13] These theories are important since they lay the foundation for understanding the complexities of the chronic pain experience, which include biological, psychological, and social influences that in turn impact pain-related function and pain-related disability.

A person's ability to work can be affected by his or her disease, disability system, and various other contextual factors. J. Elhom et al. described a step-like process starting with the person at work, then involved a disease process or injury and the subsequent complicated course to either return to work or the disability system.[14] (See Fig. 6.1.)

Models of Disability

A more complete understanding of the clinical implications of a biomedical and biopsychosocial model as it applies to pain-related loss of function and disability is imperative for the primary care provider. A biomedical model may be more applicable to acute conditions as compared to a more diverse biopsychosocial model. The biopsychosocial model may be more appropriately applied

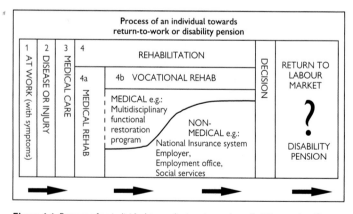

Figure 6.1 Process of an individual toward return to work or disability pension. *Source:* Reprinted with permission from Chamberlain M, Moser V, Schüldt-Ekholm K, et al. *J Rehabil Med* 2009;41:856–869. Modified after Ekholm J, et al. *Report to Ministry of Social Welfare.* Mid Sweden University, Östersund, CSF Reports No 2003:1.

to patients presenting with more chronic and disabling pain conditions many times complicated by related affective distress (i.e., depression, anxiety), sleep disturbance, deconditioning and loss of function, and a number of potentially contributing social factors (loss of vocation, financial hardship). This section will help clarify these two important conceptual models.

The biomedical model assumes a causal relationship between a specific physical pathology and the presence or intensity of pain symptoms. It emphasizes blocking or interrupting pain pathways as a means of decreasing or eliminating disease, and in the case of pain transmission, blocking and/or eliminating pain. A biomedical model may be more advantageous in treating more acute pain states, where interventional procedures, pharmacotherapy, and surgical interventions, in isolation or combination, may lead to recovery of pain or hasten time to recovery and return to normal function.

However, the biomedical model poorly addresses related mental health issues and many more complex pain conditions remain resistant to a purely biomedical approach (i.e. chronic low back pain, neuropathic pain, and fibromyalgia).[15,16] George Engel helped to shift the thinking from a purely biomedical model of disease management to a more comprehensive biopsychosocial model of illness where the "biologic," "psychological," and "social" factors are all important focuses of care.[17] Recently, the World Health Organization (WHO) has embraced a biopsychosocial model of disability, which incorporates a dynamic interaction between the individual health condition and contextual factors.[18] (See Fig. 6.2.)

Definitions

The clinician's understanding of some important terms and how they individually reflect the patient being treated are essential to proper pain treatment. Important terms include (1) impairment, (2) disability, (3) functional limitation,

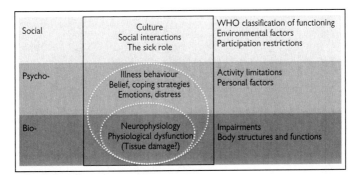

Figure 6.2 BioPsychoSocial approach. *Source:* This figure was published in Main CJ, Spanswick CC. *Pain Management: An Interdisciplinary Approach.* New York, NY: Elsevier; 2000:63–87. Copyright Elsevier 2000. Reprinted with permission.

and *(4)* handicap. *Impairment* is loss or abnormality—psychological, physical, or functional—at the level of the organs and body systems. Examples of physiologic impairments include muscle weakness, range-of-motion loss, and pain. *Disability* is a restriction or lack of ability to perform activities due to related impairments such as inability to function in a specific vocation, as a spouse, student, or parent. *Functioning* has been described as an umbrella term for body functions, body structures, activities, and participation, denoting a positive interaction between the individual or patient and contextual factors (i.e., background of the individual's life and current situation). *Functional limitation* is a deviation from the normal behavior of performing activities of daily living (ADLs) and may include problems with transfers, standing, ambulation, running, and stair climbing.[19] A formal model proposed by the International Classification of Functioning, Disability and Health (ICF) integrates the individual components into a biopsychosocial based model where a "health condition" is substituted by "chronic pain." Chronic pain is affected by body function, activities, and participation, as well as influences from the environment and personal factors.

In the last 30 years, the World Health Organization (WHO) has developed a number of models of disablement. The first included the International Classification of Impairments, Disabilities, and Handicaps (ICIDH), which included four levels of disablement: pathology, impairment, disability, and handicap. "Handicap," although a somewhat outdated term, was defined as "a disadvantage for a given individual that limits or prevents the fulfillment of a role that is normal for that individual" within their societal boundaries. The ICIDH has since been replaced by the ICF, a more comprehensive model of disablement which includes interactions between body functions and body structures, activity, and participation. The classification of these domains is affected by personal factors and environmental factors, leading to a specific, person-centered model of a health condition (disorder or disease).[20] (See Fig. 6.3.)

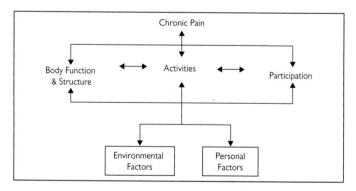

Figure 6.3 ICF Model of Disablement. *Source:* Reprinted from Weigl M, Cieza A, Cantista P, Stucki G. Physical disability due to musculoskeletal conditions. *Best Pract Res Clin Rheum.* 2007;21(1):167–190, with permission from Elsevier.

Additional important and controversial terminology pertinent to the clinician working with patients with chronic pain and pain-related disability includes *secondary gain* and *malingering*. Secondary gain, a term originally proposed by Sigmund Freud, was described as an interpersonal or social advantage attained by the patients as a consequence of being sick or having an illness.[21] In the 1970s, Finneson described secondary gain as financial rewards associated with disability. Unfortunately, clinicians may confuse the presence of potential financial rewards as equated to conscious malingering, and mistakenly assume treatment failures are due primarily to secondary gain.[22] Dersh et al. classified "internal" and "external" components of secondary gain. Examples of internal secondary gain include gratification of preexisting unresolved dependency strivings, obtaining drugs, eliciting caregiving or empathy, obtaining one's sense of entitlement after years of struggling, ability to withdraw from unpleasant or unsatisfactory life roles, or adoption of the "sick role." External gains include financial rewards (i.e., wage replacement, disability benefits, settlement), protection from legal obligations, job manipulation, or job upgrade.[23]

The clinician should also be aware of potential "losses" related to pain condition. Losses could include economic losses (overtime, take-home pay), loss of meaningfully relating to society by working, and loss of work and social relationships, recreational activities, respect, and community approval.

Many times, patient behaviors and requests for treatment, time off from work, or pain-related disability may lead the clinician to question the truthfulness of the patient's presentation. A number of terms have been used, some with negative connotations, including "symptom embellishment," "symptom magnification," and "malingering." Symptom embellishment and magnification may include a conscious or unconscious act of the patient to convince the clinician that he or she is experiencing pain or pain-related suffering. "Malingering" has been more specifically defined to include the willful, deliberate, and fraudulent feigning or exaggeration of symptoms.

Disability Programs

Multiple types of disability exist, including state and federal workers' compensation, private and disability, and Social Security. The Federal Employees' Compensation Act (FECA), the workers compensation law covering federal civilian employees and their dependents, provides continuing income maintenance payments during times of wage loss secondary to disability caused by injury at work. Medical care, benefits, and benefits from survivors are adjudicated and paid for by the federal government.

Social Security Administration Disability Programs

The Social Security Act provides cash benefits to individuals with disabilities, including both physical and mental disorders. Two major programs include the Supplemental Security Disability Insurance (SSDI) and Social Security Income (SSI). SSDI program is designed to protect those with a recent work history in

SSA-covered employment. The SSI program is aimed at those without recent work history, and they must meet a financial needs test to receive benefits.

The definition of disability in the SSA is restrictive compared to the standards used by other countries; some foreign programs compensate those who are disabled partially or temporarily, including those who are totally and permanently disabled. According to the SSA definition, disability must include the inability to work at any "substantial gainful activity" secondary to a medically determinable physical or mental impairment and be expected to last for at least 12 months. Specific SSA criteria have evolved to include a "listing of impairments."

An individual seeking compensation files a claim for benefits at a local SSA office. Information gathered by this office usually includes medical records from the claimant's personal physician, which is then forwarded to the disability determination service (DDS) at the state level. Decisions on disability eligibility are determined by a team of examiners. Those claimants denied benefits may appeal the decision, in which case a "reconsideration" is then made by a different team of examiners. Those still denied benefits may appeal and appear in front of an administrative law judge under the auspices of the SSA. Later appeals may be made to the Appeals Council of the SSA, and finally, to the federal courts.[24,25]

Assessment Tools for Neck and Low Back Pain

Outcome measures and instruments have been developed to measure aspects of health care outcomes for physical injuries and mental illness. Global scales of function include the Medical Outcomes Study 36-item Short Form Health Survey (SF-36), a standardized patient-reported assessment.[26,27] The SF-36 is composed of 36 questions related to eight health domains (physical and social role functioning, mental health, general health perceptions, vitality, and bodily pain). A short form of the some tool, the SF-12, includes a subset of 12 questions, which yields two summary scores, physical and mental health. The Pain Disability Index (PDI) is a brief measure of pain-related interference and role functioning. The PDI includes seven items rated on a 10–0nt Likert Scale (0 = no disability to 10 = total disability) assessing *(1)* family/home responsibilities, *(2)* recreation, *(3)* social activity, *(4)* occupation, *(5)* sexual behavior, *(6)* self-care, and *(7)* life support activity.

Neck and Low Back Pain-Specific Measures

The neck disability index (NDI), originally developed to assess whiplash injury, is a commonly used questionnaire for the measurement of neck pain disability and is based on the evaluation of daily living activities.[28] The NDI includes 10 questions (7 examine functional activities, 2 symptoms, and 1 concentration).

The Neck Pain and Disability Scale (NPAD) was developed to provide clinicians with the ability to assess the multidimensional effects of neck pain conditions,[29] consisting of 20 questions relating to four domains (neck function, pain intensity, emotion/cognition, and activities of daily living). The Oswestry Disability Questionnaire (ODQ) was developed to measure functional status in persons with low back pain and is a self-report measure focusing on the degree of interference in 10 functional categories, including sleep, lifting, and traveling.[30] The Roland-Morris Disability Scale contains 18 questions focusing on a patient's activity, pain, dependence on others, and emotional status.[31] A change of 2–3 points on the Roland-Morris is considered clinically significant.[32]

Disability Treatment Spectrum of Care

The treatment of patients with acute and chronic pain includes a wide spectrum of care. Most acute pain conditions may require medical management and observation. Patients may be referred for individual therapy such as physical and occupational therapy as part of an acute or chronic pain rehabilitation treatment program. Those patients who continue to report pain, decreased function, and are unable to return to previous level of work may require more formalized behaviorally based rehabilitation programs, which include work conditioning and work hardening. This section will review basic components of the work rehabilitation programs, including an overview of functional capacity testing and its utility to determining level of disability or return to work strength level.

Work Rehabilitation: Work Conditioning and Work

Work conditioning (WC) and work hardening (WH) are important core components of work therapy in the field of industrial and pain rehabilitation. This field of modern occupational therapy developed after World War II when functional rehabilitation of wounded veterans became a means to securing employment in the civilian world after returning from duty. Work therapy now includes acute treatment, job analysis and placement, and functional capacity evaluation. Multidisciplinary principles were applied to occupational therapy–based work rehabilitation in the 1950s, with the development of improved assessment tools and systems, and the addition of vocational counseling, medical management, and industrial engineering. In the 1970s, work hardening and conditioning programs were incorporated into behavioral medicine approaches with a focus on reducing abnormal illness behaviors through more comprehensive treatment of injured workers, primarily those with low back pain. Increased adoption led the Commission on Accreditation of Rehabilitation Facilities (CARF) to establish standards by the late 1980s, which were subsequently updated in the early 1990s. Work rehabilitation usually begins once a patient has reached a treatment plateau in active physical therapy and is unable to return to work due to pain-related impairments. Work rehabilitation includes structured programs that incorporate impairment related exercise, aerobic training, education, and work activity. (See Table 6.1.).

Table 6.1 Work Rehabilitation

Musculoskeletal exercise	Stability–mobility
	Strength–endurance
	Balance–coordination
Aerobic training	Equipment based
	Aerobic classes
	Functional activities
Education	Principles
	Technique training
	Problem solving
Work activity	Simulated activity
	Actual equipment
	Actual work

Source: This table was published in Demeter SL, Andersson GB. *Disability Evaluation.* 2nd ed. New York, NY: Elsevier; 2003:769–780. Copyright Elsevier 2003. Reprinted with permission.

Work conditioning is usually concentrated on the physical components of flexibility, strength, coordination, and endurance, and involves one discipline of treatment (i.e., physical or occupational therapy). A more multidisciplinary approach is seen with work hardening, which incorporates behavioral and vocational components with a formal focus on return to job-specific tasks or positions. WC is routinely coordinated with acute medical management as compared to WH, which is usually provided later in therapy within the rehabilitation phase of treatment.

Work hardening programs were initially described by Matheson as a work-oriented program focused on improvement in the "client's" productivity rather than symptom reduction or increased physical capacity.[33] A "client" can be described as an injured worker with impairments that do not match his or her job position, a worker with disease-based impairments with diminishing physical capacity, a job applicant who may not have the physical abilities to perform the intended job, or a currently employed worker in transition to a job requiring higher physical function.[34]

Work hardening is an individualized, work-specific, multi- and interdisciplinary program centered primarily on returning patients (i.e., the injured worker) to their previous level of work or work demands. WH uses real or simulated work tasks and progressively increasing conditioning, flexibility, neuromuscular control, and tolerances. Goals of WH include *(1)* attaining optimal physical tolerances and abilities, *(2)* maximizing cognitive and psychosocial functioning, *(3)* developing appropriate worker behaviors, *(4)* reducing fear and increasing confidence for resumption of productive work, and *(5)* identifying problems that may necessitate placement in an alternative job.[35,36]

An individualized WH program incorporates a three-step process, which includes an initial formal job analysis to determine specific duties, completion of a baseline work tolerance evaluation, and establishment of the individual

Table 6.2 Individualized Work Hardening Program		
Step I	**Step II**	**Step III**
Job Analysis	**Establishing Work Tolerance Baseline**	**Individual Work Hardening Plan/ Goals**
Understand worker's specific job requirements: Critical job tasks Physical job demands Psychosocial demands High-risk job factors *If job analysis available: review and validate primary job functions *If job analysis not available: on-site job task analysis	• Medical history • Worker interview • Job description with critical job demands • Pain assessment • Physical assessment • Work posture and mobility • Strength, sensation, coordination • Lifting, reaching, carrying • Pushing and pulling • Stooping, bending, kneeling • Sitting and standing • Work task stimulation	1. Increase duration of daily participation 2. Increase physical tolerances to the level of critical job demands 3. Improve body mechanics and postures 4. Develop pain management strategies 5. Develop problem-solving skills for self-management at the work site 6. Facilitate appropriate worker behaviors

Source: Work Hardening Program Standards. Washington State Department of Labor and Industries.

WH plan (see Table 6.2). WH standards have been established by a number of groups and may vary depending on state of federal governing body.

WH Program Standards

1. Improve strength and endurance in relation to return-to-work goal
2. Simulation of critical work demands, tasks, and environment to which the worker will return
3. Education: body mechanics, pacing, safety, and injury prevention, promoting worker responsibility and self-management
4. Assess for need for job modifications, that is, equipment changes or additions, ergonomic modification; availability for on-site job modification assessments
5. Individualized written plan that includes observable and measurable goals
6. Safe work or therapy environment that is appropriate for reaching vocational goals
7. Quality assurance system, outcomes based on program and worker goals
8. Documentation or reporting system that includes initial plan, regularly scheduled team conference notes with monitoring of progress, record of attendance, and compliance

9. Evaluation and modification of work behaviors, that is, timeliness, attendance, interpersonal relationship
10. Criteria for admission include physical recovery sufficient to allow for progressive reactivation and participation for a minimum of 4 hours a day for 3–5 days a week along with a defined work goal
11. Criteria for discharge clearly stated, that is, patient met goal stated in plan, patient did not participate according to program plan, goals not feasible to attain

(*Source:* Work Hardening Program Standards. Washington State Department of Labor and Industries)

Occupational therapy manages most work conditioning and work hardening treatments as part of the pain rehabilitation program. Assessment of the injured worker requires a more comprehensive one above the standard OT evaluations. Patients are placed in programs a set number of days, usually 4–5 days per week over a 4- to 8-week period. Both programs are highly based on objective measures obtained during the program evaluation, which includes tolerances and capacities for lifting, pulling, standing, sitting, reaching, climbing, kneeling, and/or crawling. The treatment program is based on the individual patient's own job demands and work level (sedentary, light, medium, heavy), and it is aimed at developing improved conditioning and tolerances for activities. (See Table 6.6.) Although formal psychological counseling is not a core discipline, these programs are based on helping patients work through and unlearn fear avoidance beliefs and abnormal or compensated movement patterns, and decrease pain-related fear and pain-related anxiety.

Functional Capacity Assessment

Functional capacity assessment (FCA) provides a means of measuring function by obtaining objective and subjective data with performance-based testing. Traditionally, health care providers can review an individual's medical history, medical records including diagnostic testing, and/or perform a physical exam to determine the level of physical impairment. These indirect measures may inaccurately quantify physical disability. More formal testing that includes across-the-spectrum FCA may help improve and more directly quantify a patient's level of function and increase chances of successful return-to-work outcomes. Testing can involve examining specific "functional units" or isolated parts of the body (i.e., lumbar spine, elbow, shoulder) or the ability of the functional unit to work with other parts of the body, examining a specific activity, commonly including lifting capacity. Lifting capacity includes the combination of movements to perform tasks. For example, a simple lifting task may include transferring forces from the hands through the elbow and more proximal shoulder, turning, flexing, and extending the lumbar spine and hips, such as transferring a container from the floor to a countertop.

Functional Capacity Testing

Functional capacity evaluation (FCE) is a process whereby the individual's ability to perform a specific task or perform a specific physical demand (i.e. sedentary, light, medium, and heavy) is assessed. And FCE helps to link patient-specific physical impairments to work capacity. Matheson describes an FCE as "a systematic method of measuring an individual's ability to perform meaningful tasks in a safe and dependable basis."[37] The purpose of an FCE includes improving the likelihood that the worker will be safe at a job, improve performance, by assessing and identifying functional problems that may be amenable to physical or occupational therapy or instruction, and to determine more objective evidence of a disability. Legal or bureaucratic entities may use this information and data to determine more quantifiable levels of impairment or apportionment for an injury or job-related condition, and/or deny or award monetary benefits.[39]

Although the primary care physician may feel uneasy managing work-related issues, including ordering or recommending restrictions, supporting requests, or disagreeing to assist a patient in his or her pursuit for short- and long-term disability, knowledge of basic principles of disability management can make this process easier and help assist the patient when appropriate. The FCE is a valuable tool for the physician and other health care providers by using more objective and validated testing measures. The primary care provider can help to determine when the patient is ready to return to work, whether restrictions are necessary, and potentially help limit recurrence of injuries after helping the patient receive proper therapy and instruction.[38,39]

Various types of FCEs can be performed by the occupational therapists (see Table 6.3.) FCEs can focus on simulating a specific vocational goal or activity, establishing goal setting, quantifying a disability rating, job matching, or more specific work capacity evaluation.[40] The time of an FCE can vary from 2 to 3 hours to 1 full workday (8 hours) or multiple days (i.e., two 8-hour sessions) and can be performed before initiation of formal therapy, repeated over the duration of therapy at time intervals where a patient may have plateaued in treatment, or at the end of the treatment to formalize strength level and plan return to work. Tests may include consideration of preinjury patient-specific baseline function or compare to validated norms. A critical part of the FCE includes validity testing, identifying any problems with patient effort and patient inconsistencies at tasks (i.e., testing a specific task as lifting a certain weight in multiple ways, self-limiting behavior, pain behaviors, and verbal reports of pain). Multiple observations, testing in specific tests, and validity testing help the therapist also

Table 6.3 Types of Functional Capacity Testing

- Establishing functional goal testing
- Disability rating
- Job and occupation matching
- Work capacity evaluation

to determine whether the test was "valid" or "invalid." Performance reliability is used to determine performance credibility based on the assumption that an individual will produce similar outcomes in a series of trials and is a key component of determining "validity."[41] Objective measures may also include increase in heart rate during and immediately following performance of a task. Performance credibility can be subjectively determined by assessing for consistency and inconsistency between specific tasks and tests.[42]

The formal finding on an FCE is usually incorporated into a more comprehensive statement that includes a level of return to work and recommendations of any type of restriction or accommodation.

Subjective credibility measures may include the individual's perceived physical strain or effort and may be rated on perceived exertion scales allowing the evaluator to better understand the individual's perception of the degree of difficulty in performing specific job-related tasks. For example, in one test, scores range from 6 to 19 (e.g., 6 [no exertion], 7 ["very, very light"], 15 ["hard"], to 19 ["very, very, hard"]) (see Table 6.4) and increase linearly with exercise intensity. The scale correlate linearly to heart rate (0.8–0.9), ranging from 60–200 beats/ minute, which is monitored and recorded by the examining therapist.[43]

Another key FCE, regardless of underlying pain condition, is grip strength. Grip strength testing measures both hand strength and more objective test for assessing performance of maximum effort. A common test used by many clinics and mentioned in FCE reports is the Jamar hand dynamometer, a calibrated hydraulic hand dynamometer, which measures static grip strength at five grip spans. Using the hand dynamometer, multiple trials at five different positions

Table 6.4 Rating of Perceived Exertion

6	
7	very, very light
8	
9	very light
10	
11	fairly light
12	
13	somewhat hard
14	
15	hard
16	
17	very hard
18	
19	very, very hard

Source: Reprinted with permission from Borg GAV. Psychophysical bases of perceived exertion. Med Sci Sports Exer. 1982;14:377–381.

are completed. The coefficient of variance is calculated. Some studies show that a number of coefficients of variance above a cutoff point indicate less than full effort. Furthermore, the score distribution will indicate maximum effort if it represents a bell curve over a span of the five different grip positions. The lowest grip force values occur in positions one and five and the highest at positions two, three, or four. Those tests results that do not produce this bell-shaped curve could cast doubt on the individual's sincerity of full maximal effort, and compared to normative values, noncredible performance.[44]

Cardiovascular endurance may also be assessed to determine whether the patient has the aerobic capacity to meet specific job demands. Endurance demands have been formally classified in the Dictionary of Occupational Titles where one MED, or metabolic equivalent, corresponds to the oxygen consumption of an individual at rest. Cardiovascular endurance may be more important specifically with patients who have related medical comorbidities (e.g., hypertension, congestive heart failure, obesity). Calculated METs ranges for specific levels of work can be assessed during formal testing (see Table 6.5.).

Functional Capacity Testing Utility

An important and controversial area of FCE results lies in its ability to demonstrate validity, reliability, and accuracy.[45,46] Results of a functional capacity test can be used in conjunction with a more detailed understanding of the individual's job description, symptoms, and tolerability for specific activity as a means of more accurately establishing return to work restrictions and formal levels of work.[47]

Primary care providers can more informally assess whether a patient is able to return to a specific level of work or job based on an informal interview and the clinician's own understanding of the relationship between physical factors, tissue pathology, and work requirement during normal work duties. Besides a specific job description, most work positions can be classified as sedentary, light, medium, heavy, or very heavy duty strength level based on U.S. Department of Labor Guidelines (see Table 6.6).

What Does an "Invalid" Test Mean?

FCE testing most importantly gives an objective overall rating of "valid" or "invalid." An "invalid" test result may be related to the patient demonstrating less

Table 6.5 Endurance Demands for Specific Work Demands	
Sedentary	1.5–2.1 METs
Light	2.2–3.5 METs
Medium	3.6–6.3 METs
Heavy	6.4–7.5 METs
Very Heavy	Over 7.5 METs

CHAPTER 6 Disability Management in Primary Care

67

Table 6.6 Classification of Work Based on Physical Demands

Physical Demand	Occasionally	Frequently	Constantly
Sedentary duty	Lift or carry up to 10 lb	Negligible	Negligible
	Sit 6–8 hr	—	—
	Stand or walk 0–2 hr	—	—
Light duty	Lift or carry up to 20 lb	Up to 10 lb	Negligible
	Stand 4–8 hr	—	—
	Walk 0–4 hr	—	—
Medium duty	Lift or carry up to 50 lb	Up to 20 lb	Up to 10 lb
	Stand or walk 8 hr	—	—
Heavy duty	Lift or carry up to 100 lb	Up to 50 lb	Up to 20 lb
	Stand or walk 8 hr	—	—
Very heavy duty	Lift or carry over 100 lb	Over 50 lb	Over 20 lb
		—	—

Source: U.S. Department of Labor. Dictionary of Occupational Titles. Washington, DC: U.S. Government Printing Office; 1986.

than full or maximum effort in performance. Although not always consistent with malingering, a number of other causes (i.e., physical ability, disability, and pain intensity) have been identified and should be considered when interpreting and making clinical decisions when a test is found to be invalid.[48,49,50]

The result of an FCE can have far-reaching consequences for injured workers, including compensation termination, job loss, or reduction in medical-legal settlement in patients believed to be exhibiting submaximal effort. To establish an objective functional capacity rating, the injured worker must perform at his or her maximal ability or effort. A number of tests have been used as a means of recording and validating effort. Other methods used to assess sincerity of effort include expected temporal relationship between heart rate changes with associated increased activity and pain reports, presence of Waddell nonorganic signs (i.e., pain in spine with axial loading, overreaction with light palpation in the skin, change in physical findings with distraction with repeat testing), overreaction and high pain behavior during testing, and grip strength measurement inconsistencies as discussed earlier.[51] (See Table 6.7.)

Summary

Primary care providers hold an important role in treating patients with acute and chronic neck and low back pain. More important, they are in a unique and important position to help identify barriers to improving outcomes, decreasing the risk for the patient developing chronic pain. The primary care provider can help patients in a number of ways such as pain-related impairments, disability, function, and quality of life. Acute pain conditions may require a more standard biomedical model. More chronic and disabling conditions require a more

Table 6.7 Causes of Invalid Functional Capacity Evaluation Tests/ Less Than Full Effort

1. Malingering syndrome
2. Factitious disorder
3. Learned illness behavior
4. Conversion disorder, pain disorder, or other somatoform disorders
5. Depressive disorders
6. Test anxiety
7. Fear of symptom exacerbation or injury
8. Fatigue
9. Medication and psychoactive substance effects
10. Lowered self-efficacy expectations
11. Need to gain recognition of symptoms

Source: American Institutes for Research. *Synthesis of Research and Development of Prototypes for a New Disability Determination Methodology: Measurement Concepts and Issues Relevant to the Social Security Administration's Disability Determination Process.* Washington, DC: American Institutes for Research; 1999.

comprehensive, pragmatic, biopsychosocial model as a means of identifying and treating tissue-related impairment, psychological factors, and social issues related to an individuals pain (i.e., family and work dysfunction). Various global and disease-specific tools are available, including the SF-12, Neck Disability Index, Oswestry Disability Questionnaire, and Roland-Morris Questionnaire.

The primary care provider, serving as a gatekeeper to patient care, may have to make important decisions regarding assisting or counseling patients with chronic pain or other chronic medical conditions that may be pursuing perma- nent disability via private insurance, state, or federal programs. Besides a thor- ough history, physical exam, and clinical workup, the clinician needs to become familiar with the basic intricacies of the disability system, including SSI and SSDI. Many times, referral to a specialist, including surgical specialists or pain man- agement clinicians, may help to better coordinate and treat these complicated clinical and administrative issues.

Pain and disability rehabilitation may include standard individual nonpharma- cologic, interventional, and behaviorally based treatment or more structured work conditioning, work hardening, or interdisciplinary functional restoration treatment programs. Disability evaluation includes more indirect methods, pri- marily including reviewing records, interviewing the patient, and physical exam- ination as compared to more formal functional capacity assessments (FCAs) and structured functional capacity evaluation (FCE). The primary care provider is encouraged to include the help of referring specialists such as pain manage- ment, occupational medicine, physical medicine and rehabilitation specialists, orthopedic surgery, and allied health professionals (i.e., physical and occupa- tional therapists, and speech pathology) in more difficult cases where disability determination and work restriction issues arise.

References

1 Field M, Jette A, eds. *Committee on Disability in America. The Future of Disability in America.* Washington, DC: Institute of Medicine of the National Academies; 2007.

2 Makela M, Heliovarra M, Sievers K, et al. Prevalence, determinants, and consequences of chronic pain in Finland. *Am J Epidemiol.* 1994;1001(124):1356–67.

3 Guez M, Hildinnsson C, Nilsson M, Toolanen G. The prevalence of neck pain. *Acta Ortho Scand.* 2001;73:455–459.

4 Clair D, Edmonston S, Allison G. Variability in pain intensity, physical and psychological function in non-acute, non-traumatic neck pain. *Physiother Res Int.* 2004;9:43–54.

5 Cleland JA, Childs J, Whitman J. Psychometric properties of the neck disability index and numeric pain rating scale in patients with mechanical neck pain. *Arch Phys Med Rehab.* 2009:89:69074.

6 Vernon H, Guerriero R, Kavanaugh S, et al. Psychological factors in the use of the neck disability index in chronic whiplash patients. *Spine.* 2009;35:E16-E21.

7 Lea R, Etheredge G, Freeman JN, Lloyd Wax B. Familial disability patterns in individuals with work-related spine injury/illness. *Spine.* 2003;28:2292–2297.

8 Bradley WG. Low back pain. *Am J Neuroradiol.* 2007;28:990–992.

9 Dagenais S, Caro J, Haldeman S. *Spine.* A systematic review of low back pain cost of illness studies in the United States and internationally. 2008;8:8–20.

10 Stanton TR, Henschke N, Maher CG, et al. After an episode of acute low back pain, recurrence is unpredictable and not as common as previously thought. *Spine.* 2008;33:2923–2928.

11 Gurcay E, Bal A, Eksioglu E, Hasturk AE, Gurcay AG, Cakci A. Acute low back pain: clinical course and prognostic factors. *Disabil Rehabil.* 2009;31:840–845.

12 Melzack R, Wall P. Pain mechanisms: a new theory. *Science.* 1965;150:971–979.

13 Melzack R. From the gate to the neuromatrix. *Pain.* 1999;6:S121-S126.

14 Ekholm J. *Report to Ministry of Social Welfare, Med Sweden University, Ostersund.* CSF Reports No 2003:1.

15 Pransky G, Shaw WS, Franche R, Clarke A. Disability prevention and communication among workers, physicians, employers, and insurers: current models and opportunities for improvement. *Disabil Rehabil.* 2004;26:625–634.

16 Carragee EJ. Persistent low back pain. *N Engl J Med.* 2005;352:1891–1898.

17 Engel GL. The need for a new medical model: a challenge for biomedicine. *Science.* 1977;196:129–136.

18 World Health Organization. *International Classification of Functioning, Disability and Health.* Geneva, Switzerland: World Health Organization; 2001.

19 American Physical Therapy Association. The guide to physical therapist practice, second edition. *Phys Ther.* 2001;81(1):9–746.

20 World Health Organization. *International Classification of Functioning, Disabilities and Health: ICF.* Geneva, Switzerland: World Health Organization; 2001.

21 Freud S. Introductory lectures on psychoanalysis. London: Hogarth, 1959.

22 Fishbain D. Secondary gain concept: definition problems and its abuse in medical practice. *Am Pain Soc J.* 1994;3:264–273.

23 Dersh J, Polatin P, Leeman G, Gatchel R. The management of secondary gain and loss in medicolegal settings: strengths and weakness. *J Occup Rehab.* 2004;14:267–279.

24 Osterwies M, Kleinman A, Mechanic D, eds. *Pain and Disability; Clinical, Behavioral, and Public Policy Perspective.* Washington, DC: National Academy Press; 1987.

25 Nibali KD. Social Security disability programs. In: Demeter S, Andersson G, eds. *Disability Evaluation.* St Louis, Mo: Mosby; 2003:44–62.

26 Ware JE, Snow KK, Kosinski M, et al. *SF036 Health Survey: Manual and Interpretation Guide.* Boston, Mass: Nimrod Press; 1993.

27 Andresen EM, Meyers AR. Health-related quality of life outcomes measures. *Arch Phys Med Rehabil.* 2000;81(Suppl 2):S30–S45.

28 Vernon H, Mior S. The Neck Disability Index: a study of reliability and validity. *J Manip Physiol Ther.* 1991;14:409–415.

29 Wheeler AH, Goolkasian P, Baird AC, Darden BV 2nd. Development of the Neck Pain and Disability Scale. Item analysis, face, and criterion-related validity. *Spine (Phila Pa 1976).* 1999;Jul 1;24(13):1290–1294.

30 Fairbank JC, Couper J, Davies JB, et al. The Oswestry low back pain disability questionnaire. *Physiotherapy.* 1980;66:271–273.

31 Roland M, Morris R. A study of the natural history of back pain: part I: development of a reliable and sensitive measure of disability in low back pain. *Spine.* 1983;8:141–144.

32 Patrick D, Deyo R, Atlas S, et al. Assessing health related quality of life in patients with sciatica. *Spine.* 1995;20:1899–1909.

33 Matheson LN. Work hardening for patients with back pain. *J Musculoskeletal Med.* 1993;Sept:53–63.

34 Isernhagen S, Work hardening. In: Demeter S, Andersson G, eds. *Disability Evaluation.* 2nd ed. St. Louis, Mo: Mosby; 2003:769–780.

35 Maultsy Burt C. Work evaluation and work hardening. In: Pedretti LC, Early MB, eds. *Occupational Therapy.* 5th ed. St Louis, Mo: Mosby; 2001.

36 Lindstrom I, Ohlund C, Eek C, et al. The effect of graded activity on patients with subacute low back pain: a randomized prospective clinical study with an operant-conditioning behavioral approach. *Phys Ther.* 1002;72:279–290.

37 Matheson L. Functional capacity evaluation. In: Andersson G, Demeter S, Smith G, eds. *Disability Evaluation.* Chicago, Ill: Mosby Yearbook; 1996.

38 Innes E, Straker L. A clinician's guide to work-related assessments: 1-purposes and problems. *Work.* 1998;11:183–189.

39 Gross DP, Battié. The prognostic value of functional capacity evaluation in patients with chronic low back pain: part 2. *Spine.* 2004;29:920–924.

40 Matheson LN. The functional capacity evaluation. In: Demeter SL, Andersson GB, eds. *Disability Evaluation.* 2nd ed. St. Louis, Mo: Mosby; 2003.

41 Matheson LN. "How do you know that he tried his best?" The reliability crisis in industrial rehabilitation. *Industrial Rehab Quart.* 1988;1:11–12.

42 Owens KA. Buchholz RL. Functional capacity assessment, worker evaluation strategies, and the disability management process. In: Shrey DE, Lacerte M, eds. *Principles and Practices of Disability Management in Industry.* Grand Rapids, Mich: GR Press; 1995:269–299.

43 Borg GAV. Psychophysical bases of perceived exertion. *Med Sci Sports Exerc.* 1982;14:377–381.

44 Matheson L, Carlton R, Niemeyer L. Grip strength in the disabled sample: reliability and normative standards. *Industrial Rehab Quart.* 1988;1(3).

45 Vasudevan SV. Role of functional capacity assessment in disability evaluation. *J Back Musculoskel Rehabil.* 1996;6:265–276.

46 Vlozo CA. Work evaluations: critique of the state of the art of functional assessment of work. *Am J Occup Ther.* 1993;47:203–209.

47 US Dept of Labor 1986. *Dictionary of Occupational Titles.* Washington, DC: US Government Printing Office; 1986. (See table on "Physical demand and level of job duty.")

48 Gross DP, Battié MC. Factors influencing results of functional capacity evaluations in workers' compensation claimants with low back pain. *Phys Ther.* 2005;85:315–322.

49 Gross DP, Battié MC. The construct validity of a functional capacity evaluation administered within a workers' compensation environment. *J Occup Rehab.* 2003;13:287–295.

50 Cutler RB, Fishbain DA, Steele-Rosomoff R, Rosomoff H. Relationships between functional capacity measures and baseline psychological measures in chronic pain patients. *J Occup Rehab.* 2003;13:249–258.

51 Lechner DE, Bradbury SF, Bradley LA. Detecting sincerity of effort: a summary of methods and approaches. *Phys Ther.* 1998;78:867–888.

Chapter 7

Complementary Pain Relief Methods for Back and Neck Pain

Yvonne D'Arcy

Many patients self-treat their back and neck pain with over-the-counter preparations such as gels and balms that can be rubbed on, an over-the-counter analgesic, or techniques such as acupuncture to reduce pain. Patients recognize that medical treatments and prescription medications are available, but they have a comfort level with trying to relieve pain with other types of approaches.

Types of Complementary and Alternative Medicine

Complementary and alternative medicine (CAM) is an attractive approach to pain relief for most patients. It requires no doctor's visit or prescription. CAM is defined as "a group of diverse medical and healthcare systems, practices, and products not presently considered to be a part of conventional medicine."[1] Many Americans use CAM methods to self-treat their pain with over-the-counter medications or techniques such as analgesic balms, hot and cold packs, or massage. Many of the therapies are minimally invasive such as acupuncture, or noninvasive such as heat, massage, or relaxation.

There are three terms that apply to complementary pain relief techniques.

Complementary: Techniques or additional therapies that are used in conjunction with recognized mainstream medical practices, for example, when massage is used concurrently with medication and or physical therapy for low back pain.

Alternative: This term means foregoing recognized medical therapy and using other treatments for a condition, for example, when acupuncture is used in place of medication and physical therapy for neck pain.

Integrative: A term coined by CAM practitioners to indicate the combined use of pharmacotherapy and nonpharmacologic methods for medical treatment. This term was popularized by Dr. Andrew Weil.[2]

As with any type of treatment, it is best to use those that have the best research support with proven outcomes. The National Institutes of Health (NIH) is studying alternative treatments and has a group called the National Center for

Complementary and Alternative Medicine (NCCAM) (www.nccam.nih.gov). This Web site will provide information on a large number of complementary techniques to include acupuncture, massage, vitamins, and supplements.

The four main types of CAM as defined by the NCCAM are as follows:

- Body-based therapies such as heat, massage, cold and acupuncture
- Cognitive-behavioral approaches or mind-body work, such as relaxation, biofeedback, and imagery
- Energy medicine, including Reiki and therapeutic touch (TT)
- Nutritional approaches that incorporate the use of herbs and vitamin supplements

Almost every American household has heating pads, cold wraps, analgesic balms, and other basic forms of pain relievers. In a 1997 survey, Americans reported that they made 629 million visits to CAM practitioners.[3] In Europe and Australia, about 20% to 70% of all patients use CAM therapies.[1] Many primary care practitioners do not ask about whether the patient is using CAM therapies, and only 40% of patients volunteer information on their use of CAM therapies without being asked.[1] In a 2002 survey the NCCAM determined that the most common conditions that patients used CAM to help relieve pain were as follows:

- Back pain
- Neck pain
- Joint pain
- Arthritis
- Headache[4]

Body-Based Therapies

Heat and Cold

Patients have easy access to heating pads and cold packs, and they are commonly used to relieve back and neck pain before any other type of treatment is tried. Most patients prefer heat and find it more comforting than applications of cold. A Cochrane report with low back patients indicates these therapies have limited support.[5] However, additional information demonstrates that using a heat wrap can increase functionality in this patient population.[5] Heat applications can reduce pain, relieve muscle spasms, increase circulation to the affected area, and decrease stiffness.[6]

Ice baths, cold packs, or ice massage is helpful for decreasing the pain of sprains and strains, low back pain, and muscle spasms.[6] RICE therapy (rest, ice, compression, and elevation), a commonly used variation of cold therapy, is used for treating minor injuries.[7] The cold applications work by:

- Decreasing nerve conduction
- Cutaneous counter irritation
- Vasoconstriction

- Muscle relaxation
- Reduction of local and systemic metabolic activity[6]

Both techniques should be used for short periods of time, and patients who have cutaneous desensitization should monitor the areas of application for skin damage.

Acupuncture

There are several types of acupuncture depending on what area of the world the practice is coming from. In most acupuncture practices, thin needles are inserted through the skin into acupuncture points.[6,8,9] Once the needles are in place, they are manipulated by hand or electrically stimulated to release neurotransmitters that increase pain relief.[9]

Acupuncture has been used for centuries on many different types of patients with a wide variety of physical complaints. Patients with cancer, fibromyalgia, osteoarthritis, labor pain, and dental pain are all patient populations where acupuncture has been found to be beneficial.[9,10] In a study with 570 patients with osteoarthritis receiving acupuncture, the patients in the study had improvements in function and decreased pain levels.[11]

For patients with neck pain, there is moderate evidence that acupuncture is more effective than sham controls.[12] There is also limited evidence that acupuncture is more effective for pain relief than massage.[12]

Massage

The NIH NCCAM defines massage as pressing, rubbing, and otherwise manipulating muscles and soft tissue in the body.[8] The effect of massage is thought to be the relaxation and lengthening of muscles, which allows oxygen and increased blood flow into the affected area.[8] For neck pain, massage has limited evidence for support.[13]

Chiropractic

A review of chiropractic interventions using spinal manipulation for low back pain found that spinal manipulative therapy was not superior to other types of therapy but was superior to placebo.[14] For neck and back pain, a meta-analysis reported that for acute lower back pain evidence exists for increased pain relief for short-term therapy over diathermy and mobilization. For chronic lower back pain the effect was considered to be similar to the use of a nonsteroidal medication and it compared favorably with physical therapy. Long-term, chiropractic treatment provides similar if not improved outcomes when compared to placebo, other medical treatments, back school, physical therapy, or soft tissue treatment.[15]

For acute neck pain there is insufficient evidence in the literature to make a recommendation for use or to determine a comparison to other types of therapy.[15] For long-term therapy there is limited evidence for support, but there is sufficient evidence to indicate that manipulation is superior to treatment by family physicians and physical therapy.[15] For pain relief, spinal manipulation therapy provides at most similar pain relief as high technology rehabilitative exercise.[15]

Other Types of Body-Based Therapies

Other forms of body-based therapies are not well supported by research. These therapies include:

- Magnets
- Copper bracelets

Physical therapy for reconditioning and improving balance can help maintain the mobility and functionality of older patients.[16] A regular physical therapy program has been found to reduce pain and improve mood.[16] If the program is individualized to the patient's ability, the patient should be able to perform at a level where improvements are possible.

Cognitive-Behavioral Therapy

Relaxation

There are several different types of relaxation techniques that can be used to help control pain.

- Regulating breathing can lead to decreased respiratory efforts.
- Relaxation tapes
- Relaxation exercises

Relaxation techniques are helpful for pain relief.[17] These techniques result in the reduction of physical tension, muscle relaxation, and the promotion of emotional well-being.[6,8] Relaxation has been found to be helpful for patients who have chronic pain, cancer pain, or surgical pain.[9] An improved sense of well-being and higher scores on quality of life scales can be attributed to the use of relaxation.[9]

Imagery

Imagery is a form of relaxation using a mental image. Images can be created by the patient or provided by tapes if patient has difficulty developing the mental images. Some older patients are not receptive to this technique. They find it difficult to relax, provide an image, and work with the mental image to create the scenario.

The Arthritis Self Management Program (ASMP) uses some mind-body techniques.[16] These include the following:

- Education
- Cognitive restructuring
- Physical activity to reduce pain
- Problem solving
- Relaxation
- Development of communication skills to help interact with health care professionals

The benefits of this program have demonstrated reduced pain that lasted over a 4-year time period and a cost savings of 4 to 5 times the cost of the program.[11]

Other types of relaxation therapies that are recognized as effective are biofeedback, hypnosis, and meditation. Coping with chronic pain can be enhanced by the use of meditation.[11] Patient preference can be accommodated since all of the techniques have research support for their use.[2]

Energy Therapy

Energy healing is derived from the concept of Qigong, an external and internal energy that has been a part of Oriental cultures for many centuries. Newer energy therapies include Reiki, therapeutic touch (TT), and healing touch.[4] Although there are differences in the practices, there are some similarities:

- The human body has an energy field that is generated from within the body to the outer world.
- There is a universal energy that flows through all living things and it is available to them.
- Self-healing is promoted through the free-flowing energy field.
- Disease and illness may be felt in the energy field and can be felt and changed by the healing intent of the practitioner.[4]

These energy therapies can be helpful to relax the patient and provide pain relief. Two of the most commonly practiced are therapeutic touch and Reiki.

Reiki

The techniques used by Reiki practitioners were developed and taught by the Buddhist monk Mikao Usui from Japan beginning in 1914.[4] Energy practitioners use the natural energy of the universe to release blockage in specific areas of the body (chakras or energy points). In this technique, a Reiki practitioner transmits energy either long distance or by directly placing hands on the patients.[8] The flow of energy opens the blocked chakras. Studies to determine the benefit of Reiki have focused on patients with cancer. In a study with 24 cancer patients using Reiki or rest periods, the Reiki patients had a significant decrease in pain.[4] The overall benefit to the patient is the sense of relaxation the patient experiences after the Reiki session.

Therapeutic Touch

The premise of TT is that the practitioner's healing force transfers or channels energy, positively affecting the recovery of the patient.[8] As the TT practitioner allows his or her hands to move over the patient, blocked energy is identified and healing forces are directed to the area to promote healing and pain relief.

There are some studies that indicate greater pain relief with the use of TT in patients with chronic pain and fibromyalgia when compared to patient groups not receiving the energy treatment option.[4] However, since a randomized placebo-controlled study is not possible with TT, it is difficult to measure the true effect of the practice.

Nutritional Approaches

Herbal Supplements

Herbal remedies are some of the most common forms of complementary therapeutics.[11] Between the years of 1990 and 1997 herbal remedy use increased by 380%.[11] The annual expenditure on herbal remedies in the United States exceeds 1.5 billion dollars annually.[11]

Dietary and herbal supplements are categorized under the DSHEA Act of 1994, which requires quality, safety, and efficacy standards. Some of the most common herbal remedies used today include the following:

- *Cayenne (Capsicum).* Cayenne can be made in plasters and placed over the painful areas. Capsaicin is the active ingredient of cayenne and is compounded into a cream that is sold over the counter as Zostrix, in two strengths, 0.025% and 0.075%.[11] To use capsaicin effectively requires 3 to 4 applications per day over at least 2 weeks to see any improvement. To avoid any contamination of other areas, wearing gloves is advised when applying the capsaicin cream.
- *Devil's claw (Harpagophytum procumbens).* Can reduce pain and increase mobility in patients with osteoarthritis.[11]
- *Willow bark (Salix alba).* Short-term improvements have been seen with this herb, but consistent results have not be obtained.[11]

Nutritional Supplements

Glucosamine and Chondroitin studies have shown that a combination of the two substances can have a positive effect in pain related to osteoarthritis and a slowing of disease progression over time.[11] It will not reverse joint damage, but it will slow the progression of joint erosion.

Omega-3 fatty acids affect prostaglandin metabolism, which is turn affects the inflammatory process. Fish oil has anti-inflammatory effects in patients with rheumatoid arthritis while flaxseed oil has not had similar effect.[11]

Summary

Complementary methods for pain relief should always be used in combination with medications for pain relief. The synergistic effect of the two types of pain relief therapies can provide more pain relief than either used alone. Most of the complementary methods are benign and noninvasive and can have a positive effect. With the variety of interventions every patient should be able to find a helpful therapy to complement his or her conventional therapy.

References

1 American Pain Society. *Pain Control in the Primary Care Setting.* Glenview, Ill: American Pain Society Society; 2006.

2 O'Hara. In: Iyer P, ed. *Medical Legal Aspects of Pain and Suffering.* Tucson, Az: Lawyers and Judges Publishing; 2003.

3 Eisenberg D. In: Iyer P, ed. *Medical Legal Aspects of Pain and Suffering*. Tucson, Az: Lawyers and Judges Publishing; 2003:476–489.

4 Pierce B. A nonpharmacologic adjunct for pain management. *Nurs Pract.* 2009;34(2):10–13.

5 French SD, Cameron M, Walker BF, Reggars JW, Esterman AJ. Superficial heat or cold for low back pain. *Cochrane Database Syst Rev.* 2006;2:CD004750.

6 American Society of Pain Management Nurses. *Core Curriculum for Pain Management Nursing*. Philadelphia, Pa: WB Saunders; 2002.

7 Berry P, Covington E, Dahl J, Katz J, Miaskowski C. *Pain: Current Understanding of Assessment, Management, and Treatments*. Reston, Va: National Pharmaceutical Council; 2006.

8 National Center for Complementary and Alternative Medicine. *Expanding Horizons of Health Care" Strategic Plan 2005–2009*. Bethesda, Md: U.S. Department of Health and Human Services, National Institutes of Health; 2004.

9 Dillard J, Knapp S. Complementary and alternative pain therapy in the emergency department. *Emerg Med Clin N Am.* 2005;23:529–549.

10 American Pain Society. *Guideline for the Management of Fibromyalgia Pain Syndrome in Adults and Childre*. Glenview, Ill: American Pain Society; 2005.

11 Khatta M. A complementary approach to pain management. *Top Adv Prac Nursing eJournal.* 2007;7(1). Available at http://www.medscape.com/viewarticle/556408. [accessed on May 26, 2011].

12 Trinh K, Graham N, Gross A, et al. Acupuncture for neck disorders. *Cochrane Reviews.* 2009;1:CD004870.

13 Heraldsson B, Gross A, Myers C, et al. Massage for mechanical neck pain. *Cochrane Database Syst Rev.* 2006;(1):CD004871.

14 Assendelft W, Morton S, Yu E, Suttorp MJ, Shekelle P. Spinal manipulative therapy for low back pain (Cochrane Review). *Cochrane Database Syst Rev.* 2004;3:CD000447.

15 Bronfort G, Haas M, Evans RL, Bouter LM. Efficacy of spinal manipulation and mobilization for low back pain and neck pain: a systematic review and best evidence synthesis. *Spine.* 2004;4(3):335–356.

16 American Pain Society. *Guideline for the Management of Pain in Osteoarthritis, Rheumatoid Arthritis, and Juvenile Chronic Arthritis*. Glenview, Ill: American Pain Society; 2002.

17 Cole BH, Brunk Q. Holistic interventions for acute pain episodes: an integrative review. *J Holistic Nurs.* 1999;17(4):384–396.

Chapter 8

Medications for Neck and Low Back Pain

Bill McCarberg

Most patients self-treat prior to seeking medical attention. Over-the-counter analgesics, including acetaminophen, aspirin, ibuprofen, and naproxen, are popular medications. Patients also use topical ice, heat, gels, creams, and braces to relieve the pain. Chiropractic treatment and acupuncture as well as herbal therapy are very common.

When a patient first presents to the provider's office, treatment has great variability. One survey of primary care physicians indicated that nonsteroidal anti-inflammatories (NSAIDs) were the most common treatment (34.7%) followed by NSAIDs plus a muscle relaxant (24.2%).[1] Results from another survey indicated that 72.4% of physicians prescribed acetaminophen, 97.7% prescribed NSAIDs, and 90.8% prescribed muscle relaxants for acute back pain.[2] This same survey found 44.8% prescribed oral steroids and 23.0% prescribed antidepressants for this condition. Much treatment for back and neck pain is not consistent with treatment guidelines. Of 720 physicians surveyed, 25% provided guideline-concordant treatment for back pain with or without radicular symptoms.[3] This variability in care may be related to the common belief among primary care physicians that they are well trained to manage back and neck pain.[4]

Only limited evidence supports the use of most medications, however. Medications can afford significant pain relief and improved function but can also be costly and have side effects. Balancing the risks and benefits requires careful consideration in patients, especially when combining drugs often taken for long periods of time and with a possibility of addiction.

A recent review by the American College of Physicians and the American Pain Society examined evidence-based guidelines for the evaluation and treatment of acute and chronic back pain.[5] This extensive treatise provides valuable information useful for the practicing clinician. Similar guidelines do not exist for neck pain. Figure 8.1 includes the management algorithm with nonpharmacologic and pharmacologic treatment recommendations. Table 8.1 is a summary of the pharmacologic treatment, shown here for easy reference. Each medication is also reviewed separately emphasizing common concerns about a specific drug or drug class.

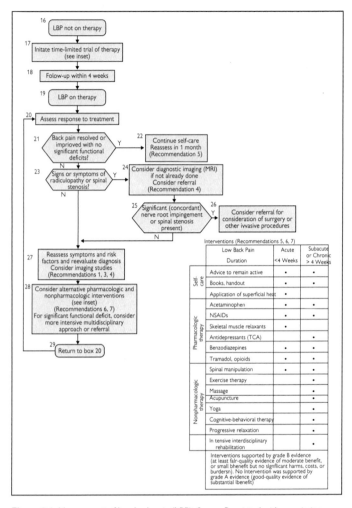

Figure 8.1 Management of low back pain (LBP). *Source:* Reprinted with permission from Chou R, Qaseem A, Snow K, et al. Diagnosis and treatment of low back pain: a joint Clinical Practice Guideline from the American College of Physicians and the American Pain Society. *Ann Intern Med.* 2007;147:478–491.

Table 8.1 Pharmacologic Treatment

Drug Class	Generic	Brand	Side Effects	Special Notes
	Acetaminophen	Tylenol	Hepatic toxicity	4 grams a day; generally safe
Nonsteroidal anti-inflammatory	Ibuprofen, naproxen, celecoxib	Motrin, Naprosyn, Celebrex	Gastric, renal, cardiovascular	Morbidity and mortality higher than any other medication class
Tricyclic antidepressants	Amitriptyline, desipramine	Elavil, Norpramin	Dry mouth, orthostatic hypotension, prolonged QT interval	Care in over 65 years old
Anticonvulsants	Gabapentin, pregabalin	Neurontin, Lyrica	Dizziness, sleepiness, cognitive impairment	No drug–drug interactions
Skeletal muscle relaxants	Cyclobenzaprine, metaxalone, Diazepam	Flexeril, Skelaxin, Valium	Sedation	Variable mechanisms of action and side effects
Opioids	Hydrocodone, oxycodone, tramadol, Tapentadol	Vicodin, Percocet, Ultram, Nucynta	Constipation, sedation, addiction	Public health concerns; may make pain worse with chronic use (hyperalgesia)
Systemic corticosteroids	Prednisone, Methylprednisolone	Solumedrol	Insomnia, osteoporosis	Very popular in clinical practice; poor trial data

Acetaminophen

Acetaminophen produces analgesia similar to aspirin, but it has no platelet effects and does not damage the gastric mucosa. Acetaminophen has very little anti-inflammatory activity, although it is a weak inhibitor of prostaglandin synthesis in vitro. The pharmacologic basis for analgesia may result from its unique ability to inhibit prostaglandin H_2 synthase.[6]

A Cochrane review of acetaminophen in acute low back pain found no difference between acetaminophen (3 g/d) and no treatment.[7] Another review examining acute and chronic back pain found no clear differences in pain relief between acetaminophen (up to 4 g/d) and NSAIDs.[8] For chronic back pain, acetaminophen was inferior to diflunisal after 4 weeks.[9]

Despite efficacy of acetaminophen in neck and back pain, its benefit is less than the nonsteroidal anti-inflammatories.[10,11] It is a reasonable first-line option for patients and can be dosed up to 4 grams a day in divided doses. Acetaminophen is often used by patients prior to seeking professional help and is perceived as weak and ineffective. Due to cost, availability, and safety, acetaminophen should be emphasized, especially at the full dose.

Although current recommendations emphasize 4000 mg/day, acute overdoses can cause potentially fatal hepatic necrosis. Unintentional overdoses occur because hidden acetaminophen is a frequent ingredient in many nonprescription and prescription analgesic formulations. The Food and Drug Administration (FDA) is currently reviewing the maximum dose recommendations due to this potential for liver toxicity. The American Geriatric Society recently reviewed acetaminophen doses in older persons and endorses the 4000 mg/day maximum.[12] Even in healthy adults, transient transaminase elevation is noted, the significance of which is unknown. Patients with chronic alcoholism and liver disease can develop severe hepatotoxicity, even at usual therapeutic doses.[13] The FDA now requires alcohol warnings for acetaminophen as well as all other nonprescription analgesics.[14]

Despite having no direct gastric mucosal effect, acetaminophen has been associated with ulcers and ulcer complications, although at a reduced risk when compared to NSAIDs. Acetaminophen is rarely associated with renal toxicity.

Nonsteroidal Anti-inflammatories

Inflammatory processes are likely occurring in acute and chronic neck and back pain. Nonsteroidal anti-inflammatories (NSAIDs) are frequently used for these pain conditions.[8] Cost also favors this drug class. A review from 24 trials found no significant differences in efficacy among drugs in the class of nonselective NSAIDs or cox-2-selective inhibitors for relief of back pain.[15] The known interpatient variability makes trials of different NSAIDs worthwhile. Despite perceived safety, well-known gastrointestinal and renovascular side effects make their use problematic. More recent cardiovascular events with the cox-2-selective agents highlight the dilemma of long-term use of this entire class. NSAIDs should be limited to the lowest effective dose for the shortest period of time.

A high-quality review by van Tulder[16] found NSAIDs superior to placebo in patient global improvement scores after 1 week of therapy. Subjects also required less breakthrough medication. For chronic low back pain, ibuprofen was also superior to placebo in one higher quality trial.[17] Another Cochrane review found no evidence of efficacy between NSAIDs and opioid analgesics or muscle relaxants, although trials were limited by small sample sizes.[18] Use of NSAIDs also was no more effective than nonpharmacologic interventions (spinal manipulation, physical therapy, bed rest).

Antidepressants

Tricyclic antidepressants (TCAs) have consistently been found to be more effective than placebo for pain relief with a small to moderate effect on pain.[19,20] Effects on functional outcomes were inconsistently reported and did not indicate clear benefits. Paroxetine and trazodone (no norepinephrine uptake effect) were no more effective than placebo. Amitriptyline is most studied and also has the most anticholinergic side effects. Caution should be observed in the elderly patient, and amitriptyline should not be used at all in patient over 65 years of age. Doses of 20–80 mg will likely be effective and full antidepressant strength is not required. Despite lack of evidence for the entire class of tricyclic antidepressants, interpatient variability recommends a treatment trial with a TCA having less anticholinergic side effects. Drowsiness (7%), dry mouth (9%), dizziness (7%), and constipation (4%) were the most common adverse events. Trials of TCA in back and neck pain were not designed to assess risks for serious adverse events, such as overdose, increased suicidality, or arrhythmias.[21]

Serotonin reuptake inhibitors show no efficacy in neck or back pain. Serotonin/norepinephrine reuptake inhibitors have been studied with duloxetine recently receiving FDA approval for chronic musculoskeletal pain, including discomfort from osteoarthritis and chronic lower back pain. Drugs in the SNRI class have indications for the treatment of depression, anxiety, diabetic neuropathy, fibromyalgia and chronic musculoskeletal pain. This class of drug will likely be effective with fewer side effects and better tolerability. Anxiety and depression are common in chronic medical illness, and the use of antidepressants for these conditions should always be contemplated.

Anticonvulsants

Multiple anticonvulsants show randomized trial benefit in a variety of neuropathic pain syndromes. Neck and back pain likely have neuropathic elements especially when the pain is chronic. Anticonvulsants are commonly used in chronic neck and back pain. Small improvements in pain compared with placebo were found in low back pain with radiculopathy using gabapentin or topiramate.[22,23] Since pregabalin has a similar mechanism of action to gabapentin, it likely would have a similar benefit as well. Other anticonvulsants either have not been studied or had negative trials in neck and back pain. Drowsiness (6%), loss of energy (6%), and dizziness (6%) were reported with gabapentin treatment.[24]

Skeletal Muscle Relaxants

Many of the studies leading to FDA approval of these drugs used small patient trials and for short periods of time.[25,26] For short-term pain in acute low back pain, a Cochrane review found skeletal muscle relaxants moderately superior to placebo relief.[27] The data are mixed on benzodiazepines.[28,29] All muscle relaxants act centrally with different mechanisms of action. There was insufficient evidence to conclude that any specific muscle relaxant is superior to others for benefits or harms.[30] Benzodiazepines will treat comorbid anxiety. Skeletal muscle relaxants were associated with central nervous system adverse events compared with placebo including sedation and fatigue, although serious complications were rare. Cyclobenzaprines carry the adverse events and warnings of the tricyclic antidepressant class of drugs. Carisoprodol (Soma) is converted by the liver into meprobamate, which has considerable dependency concerns.

Opioids

Substantial data and controversy are related to the use of opioids for noncancer pain. Analgesic efficacy is undisputed and has no rival among drug treatments. When cancer pain is evaluated, opioids are the gold standard. The cause of acute and chronic back and neck pain likely has inflammatory and neuropathic components. Two systematic reviews of placebo-controlled trials of opioids for osteoarthritis and neuropathic pain found opioids to be moderately effective.[31] In another review opioids were also superior for functional outcomes.[32] Estimates of benefit were similar for neuropathic and nonneuropathic pain. Despite a push for the use of long-acting opioids in chronic pain, there was no evidence from several trials that sustained-release opioid formulations are superior.[33,34]

Side effects are common, especially constipation and sedation.[35] Trials of opioids in low back and neck pain were not designed to assess risk for abuse or addiction and generally excluded higher risk patients. In addition, most studies were of short duration.[36] Caution must be demonstrated when prescribing opioids, due to its risk of addiction and danger to public safety as a preferred drug of abuse. Failure to establish improvements in pain or function should lead to a withdrawal of the opioid.

Tramadol is considered an opioid yet has weak activity on the μ–receptor. It likely is analgesic through a combination of μ–receptor activity and reuptake inhibition of norepinephrine and serotonin. Tramadol was more effective than placebo for chronic low back pain and functional improvement after 4 weeks of treatment.[37] No trials have compared tramadol with opioids or NSAIDs as single therapy. Withdrawal rates in clinical trials associated with adverse events were similar to placebo or the combination of acetaminophen plus codeine.[38] Nausea and dizziness result when dosages are too high, leading to intolerance.

Systemic Corticosteroids

Good-quality but small studies exist that evaluate systemic corticosteroids for acute and chronic low back pain with radicular symptoms. These studies failed to show any benefit over placebo of this treatment whether given by injection or a short oral taper.[39,40,41] Despite this lack of benefit and known side effects of treatment, oral steroid tapers are a common practice, especially with radiculopathy.

Polypharmacy

Polypharmacy has few studies sufficient to make broad recommendations. A Cochrane review comparing tizanidine with acetaminophen or a NSAID found the combination superior to either analgesic alone.[25] Clinical practice dictates that when one medication provides partial improvement in symptoms and quality of life, adding another drug with a different mechanism of action is appropriate. High-quality evidence exists using this philosophy in the treatment of hypertension and diabetes. For the physician determined to help patients suffering with neck and back pain, combining drugs may be a reasonable and rational approach despite lack of randomized trials. Combining acetaminophen, NSAIDs, skeletal muscle relaxants, and opioids may be appropriate in selected patients. When medications are combined, especially in patients already on other treatments for chronic diseases, the risk of side effects, drug–drug, and disease–drug interactions become much more likely.

Emerging Therapies

In the constantly evolving management of back and neck pain, new treatment strategies occasionally appear that may merit consideration based on mechanism of action.

Topical Nonsteroidal Anti-inflammatories

Two topical formulations of an NSAID, diclofenac, were approved by the Food and Drug Administration in 2007. Volatren Topical is a 1% gel indicated for relief of pain from osteoarthritis of joints that are amenable to topical treatment, such as the knees and the joints of the hands.[42] Flector is a 1% diclofenac preparation placed in a patch and is indicated for the topical treatment of acute pain due to minor strains, sprains, and contusions.[43] As stated earlier, the etiology of back and neck pain is often unknown yet likely has inflammatory and neuropathic components. Topical treatment has fewer side effects than orally administered NSAIDs, although no randomized trials have been done.

Duloxetine

As mentioned earlier, a newer serotonin norepinephrine reuptake inhibitor, duloxetine, recently received approval for chronic musculoskeletal pain, including discomfort from osteoarthritis and chronic lower back pain. This drug is already approved for depression, generalized anxiety disorder, diabetic peripheral neuropathy, fibromyalgia and stress urinary incontinence (Europe). Depression and anxiety are common comorbidities with chronic pain. SNRIs have favorable side effects compared to tricyclic antidepressants and should be considered in chronic back and neck pain treatment.

Nucynta

Tapentadol (Nucynta) is a new chemical compound that shows activity at the μ−receptor and inhibits the reuptake of norepinephrine. Two large randomized trials of acute pain (bunionectomy) showed pain relief similar to oxycodone.[44,45]

In another large study investigating osteoarthritis pain of the knee or hip also found comparable efficacy to oxycodone.[46] Given the dual mechanism of action, tapentadol appears similar to tramadol. Tapentadol is a much stronger opioid (schedule II) than tramadol (unscheduled) and has no serotonin activity, potentially lessening side effects. Tapentadol also does not utilize the cytochrome P450 systems, which means far fewer drug–drug interactions. One of the benefits of tapentadol appears to be fewer side effects, especially nausea and vomiting, compared to traditional opioid therapy. Tapentadol has not been studied in low back and neck pain, but opioids have shown moderate effects in these conditions. In August of 2011, the U.S. FDA approved an extended release formulation of tapentadol (Nucynta ER) for the management of moderate to severe chronic pain in adults when a continuous, around-the-clock opioid analgesic is needed for an extended period of time.

References

1 Cherkin DC, Wheeler KJ, Barlow W, Deyo RA. Medication use for low back pain in primary care. *Spine.* 1998;23:607–614.

2 Di Iorio D, Henley E, Doughty A. A survey of primary care physician practice patterns and adherence to acute low back problem guidelines. *Arch Fam Med.* 2000;9:1015–1021.

3 Webster BS, Courtney TK, Huang YH, Matz S, Christiani DC. Physicians' initial management of acute low back pain versus evidence-based guidelines. Influence of sciatica. *J Gen Intern Med.* 2005;20:1132–1135.

4 Cherkin DC, MacCornack FA, Berg AO. Managing low back pain--a comparison of the beliefs and behaviors of family physicians and chiropractors. *West J Med.* 1988;149:475–480.

5 Chou R, Qaseem A, Snow K, et. al. Diagnosis and treatment of low back pain: a joint clinical practice guideline from the American College of Physicians and the American Pain Society. *Ann Intern Med.* 2007;147:478–491.

6 Aronoff DM, Oates JA, Boutaud O. New insights into the mechanism of action of acetaminophen: its clinical pharmacologic characteristics reflect its inhibition of the two prostaglandin H2 synthases. *Clin Pharmacol Ther.* 2006;79:9–19.

7 Milgrom C, Finestone A, Lev B, Wiener M, Floman Y. Overexertional lumbar and thoracic back pain among recruits: a prospective study of risk factors and treatment regimens. *J Spinal Disord.* 1993;6:187–193.

8 van Tulder MW, Scholten RJ, Koes BW, Deyo RA. Nonsteroidal anti-inflammatory drugs for low back pain: a systematic review within the framework of the Cochrane Collaboration Back Review Group. *Spine.* 2000;25:2501–2513.

9 Hickey RF. Chronic low back pain: a comparison of diflunisal with paracetamol. *N Z Med J.* 1982;95:312–314.

10 Lee C, Straus WL, Balshaw R, Barlas S, Vogel S, Schnitzer TJ. A comparison of the efficacy and safety of nonsteroidal antiinflammatory agents versus acetaminophen in the treatment of osteoarthritis: a meta-analysis. *Arthritis Rheum.* 2004;51:746–754.

11 Zhang W, Jones A, Doherty M. Does paracetamol (acetaminophen) reduce the pain of osteoarthritis? A meta-analysis of randomised controlled trials. *Ann Rheum Dis.* 2004;63:901–907.

12 American Geriatrics Society Panel on Pharmacological Management of Persistent Pain in Older Persons. Pharmacological management of persistent pain in older persons. *J Am Geriatr Soc.* 2009;57:1331–1346.

13 Whitcomb D, Block G. Association of acetaminophen hepatotoxicity with fasting and ethanol use. *JAMA.* 1994;272:1845–1850.

14 Food and Drug Administration. *Over-the-Counter Drug Products Containing Analgesic/Antipyretic Active Ingredients for Internal Use. Required alcohol warning, CFR part 178, Docket 77N-094W.* Rockville, Md: FDA; 1998.

15 Roelofs PD, Deyo RA, Koes BW, Scholten RJ, van Tulder MW. Nonsteroidal anti-inflammatory drugs for low back pain: an updated Cochrane review. *Spine.* 2008;33:1766–1774.

16 van Tulder MW, Scholten RJ, Koes BW, Deyo RA. Non-steroidal anti-inflammatory drugs for low back pain. *Cochrane Database Syst Rev.* 2007;2:CD000396.

17 Berry H, Bloom B, Hamilton EB, Swinson DR. Naproxen sodium, diflunisal, and placebo in the treatment of chronic back pain. *Ann Rheum Dis.* 1982;41:129–132.

18 van Tulder MW, Scholten RJ, Koes BW, Deyo RA. Non-steroidal anti-inflammatory drugs for low back pain. *Cochrane Database Syst Rev.* 2007;2:CD000396.

19 Salerno SM, Browning R, Jackson JL. The effect of antidepressant treatment on chronic back pain: a meta-analysis. *Arch Intern Med.* 2002;162:19–24.

20 Staiger TO, Gaster B, Sullivan MD, Deyo RA. Systematic review of antidepressants in the treatment of chronic low back pain. *Spine.* 2003;28:2540–2545.

21 Salerno SM, Browning R, Jackson JL. The effect of antidepressant treatment on chronic back pain: a meta-analysis. *Arch Intern Med.* 2002;162:19–24.

22 Yildirim K, Sisecioglu M, Karatay S, et al. The effectiveness of gabapentin in patients with chronic radiculopathy. *The Pain Clinic.* 2003;15:213–218.

23 Khoromi S, Patsalides A, Parada S, Salehi V, Meegan JM, Max MB. Topiramate in chronic lumbar radicular pain. *J Pain.* 2005;6:829–836.

24 McCleane GJ. Does gabapentin have an analgesic effect on background, movement and referred pain? A randomised, double-blind, placebo controlled study. *Pain Clinic.* 2001;13:103–107.

25 van Tulder MW, Touray T, Furlan AD, Solway S, Bouter LM. Muscle relaxants for non-specific low back pain. *Cochrane Database Syst Rev.* 2003:CD004252.

26 Cochrane Back Review Group. Muscle relaxants for nonspecific low back pain: a systematic review within the framework of the Cochrane Collaboration. *Spine.* 2003;28:1978–1992.

27 Cochrane Back Review Group. Muscle relaxants for nonspecific low back pain: a systematic review within the framework of the Cochrane Collaboration. *Spine.* 2003;28:1978–1992.

28 Hingorani K. Diazepam in backache: a double-blind controlled trial. *Ann Phys Med.* 1966;12:125–131.

29 Moll W. Therapy of acute lumbovertebral syndromes through optimal muscle relaxation using diazepam. Results of a double-blind study on 68 cases. *Med Welt.* 1973;24:1747–1751.

30 van Tulder MW, Touray T, Furlan AD, Solway S, Bouter LM. Muscle relaxants for non-specific low back pain. *Cochrane Database Syst Rev.* 2003:CD004252.

31 Kalso E, Edwards JE, Moore RA, McQuay HJ. Opioids in chronic non-cancer pain: systematic review of efficacy and safety. *Pain.* 2004;112:372–380.

32 Furlan AD, Sandoval JA, Mailis-Gagnon A, Tunks E. Opioids for chronic noncancer pain: a meta-analysis of effectiveness and side effects. *CMAJ*. 2006;174:1589–1594.

33 Gostick N, Allen J, Cranfield R, et al. A comparison of the efficacy and adverse effects of controlled release dihydrocodeine and immediate release dihydrocodeine in the treatment of pain in osteoarthritis and chronic back pain. In: Twycross RG, ed. *The Edinburgh Symposium on Pain Control and Medical Education*. London: Royal Soc of Medicine Pr; 1989:137–143.

34 Hale M, Speight K, Harsanyi Z, et al. Efficacy of 12 hourly controlled-release codeine compared with as required dosing of acetaminophen plus codeine in patients with chronic low back pain. *Pain Res Manag*. 1997;2:33–38.

35 Hale ME, Dvergsten C, Gimbel J. Efficacy and safety of oxymorphone extended release in chronic low back pain: results of a randomized, double-blind, placebo- and active-controlled phase III study. *J Pain*. 2005;6:21–28.

36 Jamison RN, Raymond SA, Slawsby EA, Nedeljkovic SS, Katz NP. Opioid therapy for chronic noncancer back pain. A randomized prospective study. *Spine*. 1998;23:2591–2600.

37 Schnitzer TJ, Gray WL, Paster RZ, Kamin M. Efficacy of tramadol in treatment of chronic low back pain. *J Rheumatol*. 2000;27:772–778.

38 Müller FO, Odendaal CL, Müller FR, Raubenheimer J, Middle MV, Kummer M. Comparison of the efficacy and tolerability of a paracetamol/codeine fixed-dose combination with tramadol in patients with refractory chronic back pain. *Arzneimittelforschung*. 1998;48:675–679.

39 Finckh A, Zufferey P, Schurch MA, Balagué F, Waldburger M, So AK. Short-term efficacy of intravenous pulse glucocorticoids in acute discogenic sciatica. A randomized controlled trial. *Spine*. 2006;31:377–381.

40 Haimovic IC, Beresford HR. Dexamethasone is not superior to placebo for treating lumbosacral radicular pain. *Neurology*. 1986;36:1593–1594.

41 Porsman O, Friis H. Prolapsed lumbar disc treated with intramuscularly administered dexamethasonephosphate. A prospectively planned, double-blind, controlled clinical trial in 52 patients. *Scand J Rheumatol*. 1979;8:142–144.

42 Package insert for Voltaren Topical. Available at http://www.accessdata.fda.gov/drugsatfda_docs/label/2009/022122s006lbl.pdf

43 Package insert for Flector. Available at http://www.accessdata.fda.gov/drugsatfda_docs/label/2008/021234s003lbl.pdf

44 Daniels SE, Upmalis D, Okamoto A, Lange C, Häeussler J. A randomized, double-blind, phase III study comparing multiple doses of tapentadol IR, oxycodone IR, and placebo for postoperative (bunionectomy) pain. *Curr Med Res Opin*. 2009;25(3):765–776.

45 Daniels S, Casson E, Stegmann J-U, et al. A randomized, double-blind, placebo-controlled phase 3 study of the relative efficacy and tolerability of tapentadol immediate release (IR) and oxycodone IR for acute pain. *Curr Med Res Opin*. 2009;25(6):1551–1561.

46 Hartrick C, Van Hove I, Stegmann J-U, Oh C, Upmalis D. Efficacy and tolerability of tapentadol immediate release and oxycodone HCl immediate release in patients awaiting primary joint replacement surgery for end-stage joint disease: a 10-day, phase III, randomized, double-blind, active- and placebo-controlled study. *Clin Ther*. 2009;31(2):260–271.

Chapter 9

Interventional Options for Managing Chronic Back and Neck Pain

Steven Stanos and Yvonne D'Arcy

When the patient with low back pain or neck pain continues to have unrelieved pain, the health care practitioner can consider a referral to a pain clinic or pain specialist for evaluation or an interventional treatment option. When deciding which type of pain referral to make, the health care practitioner should carefully consider the type of pain that the patient has. If a patient with low back or neck pain has a radicular component to his or her pain, a good option for referral would be an anesthesia-based pain clinic where epidural steroid injections are performed regularly. Approximately 50% of patients referred to a pain clinic with neck pain have facet-related pain, which can respond very well to a facet injection.[1] If the patient has neck pain that limits motion and is painful, a rehabilitation or physical medicine clinic with a focus on physical therapy and medication management might be the best option. The key to success with a pain clinic referral is to understand the patient's pain and refer to the correct type of clinic for evaluation.

As pain clinics became popular with both patients and referring physicians, the number of pain clinics grew dramatically, numbering 1200 pain facilities by 1987, and with current numbers ranging from 2650 to 3000 (American Pain and Wellness, http://www.painandwellness.com). However, currently data indicate that there are only 6 board-certified pain specialists for every 100,000 patients.[2] This severely limits the number of patients who can be seen in these specialty clinics and accounts for the long wait patients experience when they are referred for treatment.

When Should You Refer a Patient for Interventional/ Pain Clinic Management?

Most health care practitioners tend to attempt to manage pain in their patients with a combination of medications, physical therapy, or other treatment options such as heat or cold packs. For many patients this approach will work, but only 58% of patients with chronic pain are satisfied with their analgesics.[3] This can lead to noncompliance or misuse of medications by the patient, resulting in a poor outcome. An interventional option may be needed to help relieve or decrease pain and increase functionality in patients who have failed medication therapy and still report high levels of pain.

In general, a pain clinic referral is indicated when the following occur:

- Multiple medications and doses have been tried, without good result.
- Over time the patient continues to have severe pain, making compliance with the recommended plan of care difficult (e.g., physical therapy or reconditioning).
- The health care practitioner needs confirmation that the current plan of care is the most appropriate for the patient's pain complaint.
- The pain the patient is having may be radicular in nature, which could respond well to an interventional approach such as an epidural steroid injection.

No matter what type of pain or intervention is being considered, the patient who is referred to the pain clinic will have a multidimensional pain assessment and evaluation process that will help determine just what type of treatment will benefit the patient

Common Interventional Pain Management Options

Most interventional pain clinics have the ability to perform a group of common interventional pain treatment techniques.

- Injections such as epidural steroid injections, facet joint injections
- Prolotherapy
- Radio frequency lesioning/Intradiscal electrotherapy (IDET)
- Epiduroscopy
- Spinal cord stimulators
- Implanted intrathecal pumps

After evaluating the patient, assessing the pain complaint, and the condition of the patient, the pain specialist will select an option that will provide the biggest benefit to the patient. As a part of the comprehensive pain assessment and evaluation process, the patient will need to provide information on the following:

- Medical history
- Surgical history
- Past pain experiences
- Any history of a substance abuse disorder, alcohol use, or previous illicit drug use
- Psychiatric history
- Medication use history
- Laboratory findings
- Imaging results (e.g., CT scans or MRIs)
- Other pertinent workup results (e.g., EMG[4])

Once the information is obtained and evaluated, the pain specialist will speak to the patient about what options are available and which options will best meet the patient's needs.

Spinal Injections

Some spinal injections are performed as a treatment while others are used as a diagnostic tool. Some common indications for spinal injections include the following:

- Age-related changes in the spine with bone spurs and facet arthopathy, nerve impingement, or degenerative disk disease (DDD)
- Failed back syndrome where there is still nerve impingement present
- Herniated nucleus pulposus (HNP) commonly called sciatica, where a nerve root is being compressed and radicular pain is present
- Spinal stenosis caused by a thickening of the spinal bones as they age, causing compression on the neural elements of the low back
- Cervical facet syndrome diagnosed with a combination of symptoms, including axial neck pain, pain with pressure on the affected facet joints, pain and limitation of extension and rotation, and absence of neurological symptoms[1]

These types of injections are elective and are not guaranteed to be successful. An important contraindication for injection therapy is infection or anticoagulation.[5] Some complications of ESI include psychogenic reaction, drug-related complications, needle-related injuries, and infectious complications.[6]

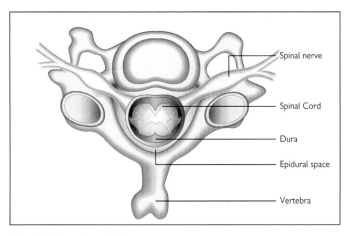

Figure 9.1 Normal vertebral structures.

Facet Injections

Facet injections are performed to relieve pain that is being generated by the zygapophyseal joint. It is caused by a loss of height or shrinking of the disk or vertebra, causing laxity in the facet joint. As with other types of injection, there is a diagnostic phase where two injections can be performed at 2-week intervals and then in the treatment phase the interval should be 4 to 6 weeks. In the case of cervicogenic headache, procedures may take place at intervals of 6 weeks after the treatment phase is completed.[7]

Cervical facet pain as defined earlier has a prevalence rate of 25% to 65% within a population suffering from neck pain.[1] Use of a diagnostic block with local anesthetic only can help confirm the diagnosis of cervical facet syndrome. The use of a cervical facet block with a local anesthetic and steroid in the intra-articular facet space can be beneficial. In a randomized controlled study with bupivacine alone or bupivacaine and steroid pain reduction lasted for 14 to 16 weeks in both groups.[1] With a very low complication rate the option of a cervical block can provide pain relief for an extended period of time, and it can be repeated.

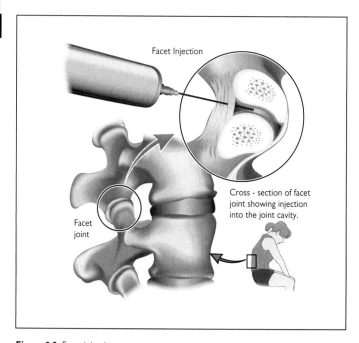

Facet Injection

Cross - section of facet joint showing injection into the joint cavity.

Facet joint

Figure 9.2 Facet injections.

Epidural Steroid Injections

Since low back pain and neck pain are common pain complaints for patients, 70% to 80% and 60%, respectively, at some point in their lifetime, many patients will be offered and receive an epidural steroid injection.[8] An epidural steroid injection (ESI) can be performed at almost any level of the spine to treat either back pain or neck pain. To perform an epidural injection, fluoroscopy is used to locate the area of pain. A newer approach to visualizing the area for injection is ultrasound. It can reduce the time to perform the block, number of attempts, and reduce block onset time.[9] Combining the use of ultrasound and fluoroscopy can provide a higher success rate than either technique when used alone.

Once the site for injection is located, a needle is then inserted through the back into the epidural space of the spinal column and a solution of local anesthetic and steroid is injected. Localized relief is provided directly at the pain stimulus.[10] All solutions used for these injections must be preservative free. The most commonly used local anesthetics are bupivacaine and ropivacaine, and depomedrol is a commonly used steroid. The effect of the injection is not immediate in most cases and it may take 5–7 days for the full effect to take place. The suggested injection interval is 1 to 2 weeks in the diagnostic phase and then 2 months if greater than 50% pain relief is achieved with the first series of injections.[7] The maximum limit for the injections is 4 to 6 times per year. In most cases preauthorization from insurance providers is required.

The four types of epidural injections recognized by the ASIPP's Systematic review include the following:

- Caudal epidural injections—strong evidence for short-term pain relief and moderate for long-term pain relief of chronic low back pain and radicular pain
- Interlaminar epidural injections—strong short-term and limited long-term pain relief for lumbar radiculopathy
- Selective nerve root injections—moderate pain relief has been demonstrated for nerve root irritation
- Transforaminal epidural injections—strong evidence for short-term and limited evidence for long-term pain relief of lumbar radicular pain[7]

The research support for these techniques is evolving. A Cochrane review , indicates no evidence for pain relief for chronic or subacute low back pain.[11] Another systematic review by Nelemans et al. indicates injection therapy did not prove to be more effective than placebo. More recently the American Pain Society's Low Back Pain Guidelines[12] had similar indications for pain relief with injection therapy. This does not mean that these techniques are not supported by outcomes, just that there is not enough strong research to support practice recommendations.

Sacroiliac Injections

When a patient has low back pain or leg pain there should be high suspicion that the sacroiliac joint is the pain generator. It has a large number of nerves that can become compressed or irritated causing low back or leg pain. Approximately

20% of back and leg pain reported to health care practitioners is caused by the sacroiliac joint, although it can easily be confused with radiculopathy.[13] The results of sacroiliac injection are found to be limited for both short- and long-term pain relief.[14]

Trigger/Tender Point Injections

If a patient can point to a painful area, a trigger point injection may be suggested to relieve the pain. Myofascial pain syndrome is one pain condition where a localized injection has shown some efficacy. To perform the procedure, local anesthetic (Lidocaine) is injected directly into the painful area. The drawback to the technique is the short-term pain relief that the injection provides. Once the local anesthetic wears off, the pain begins to return.

Botulinum Toxin (Botox) Injections

Botulinum toxins are a product of the anaerobic bacteria *Clostridium botulinum*. The FDA has approved several different botox neurotoxins for the purpose of treating the pain of cervical dystonia.[15] Intramuscular botox was identified as beneficial when used as an adjunct for relieving pain and muscle spasms of low back pain but not in whiplash associated disorders or chronic neck pain.[16] Additionally a Cochrane review indicates that a Botox injection when used alone is no better than saline at decreasing pain or improving disability.[17] With the mixed reviews, the use of Botox for pain relief should be carefully considered.

To use a Botox injection for cervical dystonia, the toxin is injected directly into a muscle with muscle weakness occurring within 2 weeks. The weakness resolves gradually as function slowly returns to normal. The effect is reported to be about 3 months. Patients have reported that the pain from an injection is higher than the blocking effect.[15] The recommended treatment interval is 12 weeks.[15]

Other conditions that are not FDA approved where Botox has been used include the following:

- Migraine headaches. Discovered as a side effect of the use of Botox for plastic surgery injections. In a study of plastic surgery patients who received Botox for cosmetic purposes, 51% of 77 patients with migraine reported complete relief of headache and 38% of 77 patients reported partial relief.[15] Other headache types that Botox has been used for include tension, cluster, and chronic daily headaches.
- Musculoskeletal pain to include chronic temporomandibular joint dysfunction, chronic cervicothoracic pain, chronic low back pain, and pyriformis syndrome.[4]

Other Therapies

There are a variety of other options that are used by interventionalists for relieving pain if more standard therapies fail to provide adequate pain relief. These options include radiofrequency lesionin; for specific muscle groups, prolotherapy may be used. Since the techniques are considered to be secondary or third-tier options, there is limited research available and support may not be strong for these techniques as a result. This does not mean the techniques have no value, just that the literature to provide research support has not yet been developed.

Prolotherapy or Regenerative Injection Therapy

The injection of an irritant solution such as dextrose/phenol/glycerine or pumice into weakened back muscles has been found to provide pain relief when combined with an aggressive physical therapy regimen.[18] There are any number of conditions where this technique has been tried, such as the following:

- Discogenic back pain
- Chronic pain form ligament or tendons form repetitive motion disorder
- Osteoarthritis
- Cervical, thoracic, lumbar, lumbosacral, and sacroiliac instability[19]

Without the physical therapy program, the technique has little evidence to support its use.

Radiofrequency Lesioning, Intradiscal Electrothermal Therapy

These therapies use a heated probe to transect the nerve in the painful area. This practice has provided anecdotal reports of pain relief for discogenic back pain. In a randomized, double-blind, controlled trial of intradiscal electrothermal therapy (IDET) versus placebo, the study findings revealed no significant benefit for the IDET patients over the placebo group.[20] However, a comparison of IDET with spinal fusion therapies demonstrated that 50% of the patients treated with IDET were able to avoid surgery.[21]

Epiduroscopy

Epiduroscopy involves the insertion of a scope into the epidural space of the spine to perform adhesiolysis. Attached to the scope are tools that can be used to remove scar tissue from nerve roots that has been found to be a source of inflammatory pain. The technique has been trialed with limited success. There is insufficient research to indicate whether the risk–benefit ration of this technique merits its use.

Implanted Modalities

Intrathecal drug delivery systems are used to control intractable chronic pain or malignant pain in patients.[14] This technique is not a first-line option and requires

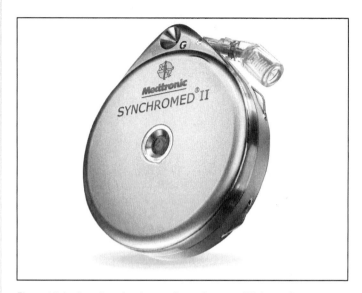

Figure 9.3 Implanted intrathecal pump. *Source:* Courtesy of Medtronic, Inc.

failure of multiple medications and dose titrations. In order to permanently place an implanted pump, a trial of the technique is performed to determine efficacy of the modality.

An implanted computerized pump automatically delivers a prescribed dose of medication at a set rate. The medication is delivered from the pump reservoir into the intrathecal space by a flexible catheter that is tunneled from the spinal insertion point along the lateral aspect of the patient's body and connected to the pump. The pump is placed into a pocket in the abdominal or other subcutaneous tissue close to the skin's surface to make refilling the pump easier.

Medications that are FDA approved for use in implanted intrathecal pumps are as follows:

- Morphine
- Baclofen
- Zinconitide (Prialt)

Using other medications than those just listed can cause pump malfunction if pump parts deteriorate. All medications used in implanted intrathecal pumps should be preservative free. Morphine is the most common medication and using an intrathecal medication delivery can provide morphine doses that are 300 times as potent as oral morphine.[5] Before the pump is permanently implanted, a trial will be performed using the anticipated medication, generally morphine. During the trial period, the drug selection is based on the following:

- History of opioid tolerance
- Side effect history
- Pain afferent spinal cord level compared with catheter tip location.[4,5]

Prialt is a one of a kind medication classed as a neuronal-type (N-type) calcium channel blocker. It is derived from the venom of the cone snail, a marine snail. Prialt must be administered intrathecally using a continuous infusion.[22] It can be used to treat both chronic and neuropathic pain.[23] There are some significant side effects, mainly neuropsychiatric. These include the following:

- Depression
- Cognitive impairment
- Depressed levels of consciousness
- Hallucinations
- Elevated creatinine kinase levels.[4,22]

Prialt use should be considered only after a trial of all other mainstream treatments. Patients who receive Prialt should be evaluated prior to use for any current psychiatric conditions that would preclude the use of the drug. They should also be carefully reassessed after the treatment begins for any signs of adverse events.

The use of an intrathecal medication delivery system can have any number of problems. The patient risk–benefit ratio should be carefully weighed and all other reasonable options should be tried before the pump implantation is tried. If during the trial the patient does not have a 50% reduction in pain levels, pump placement should be reevaluated. There is strong evidence for use of implanted pumps for short-term improvement of malignant or neuropathic pain. There is modest evidence for long-term use.[14]

Table 9.1 Selecting a Candidate for Intrathecal Medication Delivery

- Ineffective oral analgesia with multiple oral or transcutaneous trials including dose titration
- Intolerable side effects despite opioid rotation
- Functional analgesia during temporary trial infusion
- Psychological stability and reasonable goals
- Access to care: the patient will return to the pain clinic for pump refills and dose adjustments
- Patient acceptance
- For baclofen: intractable spasticity unrelieved by oral antispasmodics with improved spasticity with baclofen test dosing

Source: Reprinted with permission from Wallace M, Staats P. *Pain Medicine and Management.* New York, NY: McGraw-Hill; 2005:342.

Spinal Cord Stimulation

Spinal cord stimulation (SCS) is considered to make use of the gate control theory of pain generation and inhibition. As the pain stimulus continues to present itself to the neuron, the gate opens to transmit the pain stimulus. Spinal cord stimulation acts to selectively depolarize large fiber afferents in the dorsal columns of the spinal cord closing the gate without causing motor effect.[5] It is also considered that the sympathetic nervous system is activated by the pulse generation of the stimulator and that additional neuronal pathways may be activated and provide additional pain relief.[5] Indications for use for SCS include failed back syndrome, complex regional pain syndrome, angina, pelvis pain, and peripheral vascular disease.[14]

An implanted pulse generator, similar in size to a cardiac pacemaker, delivers electrical pulses to a lead located in the targeted spinal cord area, the area that is painful.[24] The generator is attached to a lead or leads that are implanted into the epidural space at the site of pain generation either percutaneously or through a laminectomy. When the system is activated, the patient will feel a tingling, or paresthesia, over the affected or painful area. The SCS stimulation feeling is often compared to the tingling feeling of a transcutaneous electrical nerve stimulation (TENS) unit.

The technique is a treatment option covered by Medicare and other governmental health care programs, all major commercial health plans, and most worker's compensation plans in the United States.[25] The evidence for SCS indicates that is has strong evidence for short-term pain relief of failed back

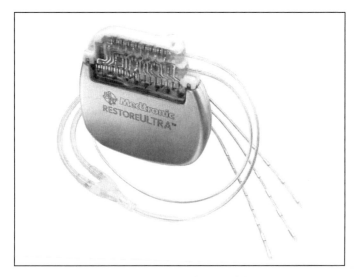

Figure 9.4 Implanted pulse generator. *Source:* Courtesy of Medtronic, Inc.

Table 9.2 Criteria for Appropriate Patient Selection for SCS
• All acceptable and less invasive treatment options should be exhausted.
• The patient should have a psychiatric evaluation to evaluate the patient for any psychiatric comorbidities, any issues of substance abuse, and any potential for secondary gain.
• A diagnosis should be established for the pain.
• Test stimulation trials indicate a good level of pain relief and functional improvement.
Sources: Neuromodulation Therapy Access Coalition (NTAC). *Position Statement on Spinal Cord Neurostimulation.* 2008; Wallace M, Staats P. *Pain Medicine and Management.* New York, NY: McGraw-Hill; 2005.

syndrome and complex regional pain syndrome with moderate evidence for long term pain relief.[7] The last positive aspect of SCS is that it is minimally invasive, reversible, nondestructive, and if the technique does not provide the expected result the lead(s) and generator can be explanted.[25]

Summary

There is a definite value in sending a patient to an interventional pain clinic for evaluation if the current pain regimen is not sufficient for effective pain relief. For patients with neck and back pain a multimodal approach including interventional options can provide optimal pain relief. Sending the patient with these conditions to a pain specialist does not mean an injection or interventional technique will be used. In some cases the original plan of care for the patient will be reconfirmed. In other cases the addition of an intervention can provide the added pain relief the patient needs to participate more fully in the plan of care and rehabilitation.

References

1 van Eerd M, Patijn J, Lataster A, et al. Evidence based medicine: cervical facet pain. *Pain Practice.* 2010;10(2):113–123.

2 Breuer B, Pappagallo M, Tai JY, Portenoy RK. U.S. board-certified pain physician practices: uniformity and census data of their locations. *J Pain.* 2007;8(3):244–250.

3 American Pain Foundation. *Pain Facts: An Overview of American Pain Surveys.* 2005. Available at: http://www2.cdc.gov/phlp/conferencecd2006/docs/hand_3.pdf [accessed on May 27, 2011].

4 D'Arcy Y. *A Compact Clinical Guide to Chronic Pain.* New York, NY: Springer Publishing; 2011.

5 Wallace M, Staats P, eds. *Pain Medicine and Management: Just the Facts.* New York, NY: McGraw-Hill; 2005.

6 Benedetti EM, Siriwetchadarak R, Stanec J, Rosenquist RW. Epidural steroid injections: Complications and management. *Techniques in Regional Anesthesia & Pain Management.* 2009;13(4):203–298.

7 Boswell MV, Trescot AM, Datta S, et al. American Society of Interventional Pain Physicians. Interventional techniques: evidence-based practice guidelines in the management of chronic spinal pain. *Pain Physician.* 2007;10(1):7–111.

8 Deer T, Ranson M, Kapurat L, Diwan S. Guidelines for the proper use of epidural steroid injections for the chronic pain patient. *Tech Reg Anesth Pain Manag.* 2009,13:288–295.

9 Shankar H. Ainer C. Ultrasound guidance for epidural steroid injections. *Tech Reg Anesth Pain Manag.* 2009;13:229–235.

10 Armon C, Argoff C, Samuels J, Backonja M. Assessment: use of epidural steroid injections to treat radicular lumbosacral pain: report of the Therapeutics and Technology Assessment Subcommittee of the American Academy of Neurology. *Neurology.* 2007;68(10):723–729.

11 Nelemans PJ, deBie RA, deVet HC, Sturmans F. Injection therapy for acute and chronic benign low back pain. *Cochrane Rev. ACP Journal* 2000;133(1):27.

12 Chou R, Huffman L. Medications for acute and chronic low back pain: a review of evidence for an American Pain Society/American College of Physicians Clinical Practice Guideline. *Ann Int Med.* 2007;147(7):505–514.

13 Maigne JY, Aivaliklis A, Pfefer F. Results of sacroiliac joint double block and value of sacroiliac pain provocation tests in 54 patients with low back pain. *Spine.* 1996;21(16):1889–1892.

14 Trescott A. Interventional approaches to the management of spinal pain: a summary of ASIPP's evidence-based guidelines. *Pain Med News.* 2009;7(12):85–95.

15 Argoff C. In: Wallace M, Staats P, eds. *Pain Medicine and Management: Just the Facts.* New York, NY: McGraw-Hill; 2005:285–288.

16 Langevin P, Lowcaock J, Weber J, et al. Botulinum toxin intramuscular injections for enck pain: a systematic review and metaanalysis. *J Rheumatol.* 2011;38(2):1–12.

17 Peloso P, Gross A, Haines T, Trinh K, Goldsmith CH, Burnie S, Medicinal and injection therapies for mechanical neck disorders. *Cochrane Database Syst Rev.* 2007;3:CD00319.

18 Yelland MJ, Del Mar C, Pirozzo S, Schoene ML. Prolotherapy injections for chronic low back pain: a systematic review. *Spine.* 2004;29(19):2126–2133.

19 Linetsky. In: Wallace M, Staats P, eds. *Pain Medicine and Management: Just the Facts.* New York, NY: McGraw-Hill; 2005:285–288.

20 Freeman B, Fraser R, Cain C, Hall D, Chappie D. A randomized, double blind, controlled trial: intradiscal electrothermal therapy versus placebo for the treatment of chronic discogenic low back pain. *Spine.* 2005;30(21):2369–2377.

21 Andersson GB, Mekhail NA, Block JE. Treatment of intractable discogenic low back pain. A systematic review of spinal fusion and intradiscal electrothermal therapy (IDET). *Pain Physician.* 2006;9(3):237–248.

22 Lynch SS, Cheng CM, Yee JL. Intrathecal ziconotide for refractory chronic pain. *Ann Pharmacotherapy.* 2006;40(7–8):1293–1200.

23 Schroeder CI, Doering CJ, Zamponi GW, Lewis RJ. N-type calcium channel blockers: novel therapeutics for the treatment of pain. *Med Chem.* 2006;2(5):535–543.

24 Mailis-Gagnon A, Furlan A, Sandoval JA, Taylor R. Spinal cord stimulation for chronic pain. *Cochrane Database Syst Rev.* 2004;3:CD003783.

25 Neuromodulation Therapy Access Coalition (NTAC). *Position Statement on Spinal Cord Neuromodulation.* 2008. Available at http://www.aapm.org

Chapter 10

Transition from Hospital to Home

Yvonne D'Arcy

When patients with chronic back and neck pain consider having surgery to correct a back or neck pain problem, there are some very important issues to consider. Many of these patients will be taking opioids, either short-acting or extended release preparations. They may also be taking these medications long term over the course of several years. In addition, they may be using other co-analgesic medications such as antidepressant or neuropathic pain drugs. This means that many will be heavily opioid dependent and have complex analgesic needs while they are hospitalized for their surgery.

Using surgery to correct neck and back conditions that are painful can be risky. There is no guarantee of success. For some patients the surgery is effective and the patient's pain is relieved. In many cases, this may be the outcome, but in other instances the back or neck pain may not improve and may even worsen. For patients for whom surgery is successful, a better quality of life is possible. For the remainder of the patients for whom surgery is not fully successful, depression may increase or the patients may feel disappointment about having an additional procedure without the benefit they had planned.

When patients with back and neck pain are considering a surgical procedure, it is important to set the right expectations. This involves a real and complete explanation of the process and a frank discussion with the patient about the potential outcomes of the procedure. By setting realistic expectations with the patient in a preoperative setting, the patient will be more relaxed and accepting when the outcome is not perfect immediately after surgery.

Patients should also consider how their chronic pain and the medications they take for pain management will affect their surgical experience. For example, patients who are taking opioids for a period of more than 4 weeks prior to surgery should expect that the amount of medication needed to control their pain after surgery will be higher and pain relief may be more difficult to achieve. This is the result of tolerance and physiologic changes, such as neuronal remodeling, NMDA activation, and wind-up, that occur when pain continues long term.

It is also important to remember that patients with long-term pain have had many experiences with the health care system. Some will have been successful, while others may have been very demeaning, for example, incidences when they may have been labeled as addicted or drug seeking. Bringing these experiences into a surgical setting can cause the patient to be cautious and distrusting of the medical system and individual providers. Building a trusting relationship requires an honest and forthright approach to questions and patient concerns.

Inpatient Issues

Patients with chronic pain are more difficult to treat for surgical pain in the postoperative setting only because there are complex pain management needs that need to be addressed.

These complex needs can include the following:

- Tolerance to opioids
- Physical dependence on opioids for chronic pain relief
- The need for higher doses of pain medication to control postoperative pain[1,2]

The American Society of Anesthesiologists has recommendations for controlling pain in the perioperative period.[3] These recommendations include the following:

- The use of opioid medications in the perioperative period
- Regional anesthesia techniques such as blocks
- The use of patient controlled analgesia (PCA) in the postoperative time period[3]

Once the back or neck surgery patient can take oral medications, the best approach is to restart the baseline medications and add additional medication to control the surgical pain. The expectation that the surgical patients will be free of pain in the postoperative time period is unrealistic. Instead, the patient should be encouraged to expect that all efforts will be made to make the pain tolerable for the patient. The goal for the patient is to become more functional; therefore, pain medication should be used to control pain to a tolerable level so that participation in physical and occupational therapy is not delayed.

Most patients with back and neck surgery have referrals for physical and occupational therapy. These services will help the patients become more able to care for themselves and participate in rehabilitation after discharge. During the postoperative recovery period, the patients will be taught helpful techniques to use at home. These include the following:

- Occupational therapy techniques to move from the bed to a chair or standing with minimal strain on the surgical area
- The appropriate way to move from bed to standing, log rolling
- How to walk with a walker or other assistive device
- The use of toilet riser to make it easier for the patient to lower to the toilet
- The use of assistive devices such as reachers for patients with limited mobility

- Exercises to help strengthen the neck or back muscles and increase mobility, flexion, extension

The ability of the patient to function in physical therapy and participate fully in twice per day sessions is crucial to helping determine the type of discharge planning that is needed. To achieve the best outcome, the patient will need adequate pain control and the desire to help in his or her rehabilitation process. For patients with back and neck pain this may not be an easy task since they may have been less active prior to surgery and are coming in for surgery in a deconditioned state. It is extremely important for the patient to take an active role in the entire rehabilitation process.

   To progress to discharge, patients are encouraged to walk and move around the hospital unit if they are able. Staying in bed and continuing to use intravenous pain medication for many days is discouraged. As soon as possible, the use of intravenous opioids is discontinued with the main pain relief coming from oral preparations. The patient's baseline medication doses may have to be temporarily increased, but they should be able to titrate to lower levels as the surgical pain resolves and the full results of the surgery are felt.

Discharge Planning

When planning a patient's discharge, postoperative back and neck pain patients may have options that are limited by insurance and their ability to participate in physical and occupational therapy. If they are severely deconditioned and unable to fully participate, they may need to go to a higher level of care on discharge. Although there may be many different facilities for rehabilitation of back patients, for those who are not able to participate in full therapy sessions in the hospital, a skilled nursing facility may be the option needed, though not really the one the patient prefers. The social services or discharge planning specialists in the hospital will review each patient's insurance coverage and help each patient with placement and discharge needs.

   There are four basic types of placements that are available for postoperative back and neck patients when they are discharged:

- Skilled nursing facility (SNF)—This option is for patients who cannot tolerate a full physical and occupational therapy regimen. The physical therapy in this setting is approximately 1 hour per day.
- Acute rehabilitation facility—The requirement for participation in physical and occupational therapy is 3 hours per day. It is more likely that this placement option would be chosen for a patient who has comorbidities that make home placement too difficult.
- Home with home care—This option has a home physical and occupational therapy option three times a week.
- Home with outpatient therapy—This option provides for placing the patient in his or her home with attendance at an outpatient physical and occupational therapy program for therapy sessions several times a week.

The reimbursement for these services may vary from state to state and with the different types of insurance. With the narrowing coverage and changes in criteria for patient placement, home placement is becoming more frequent even with significant surgical procedures.

Physical therapy and rehabilitation may take many months. The patient may never be able to discontinue the strengthening exercises and may need to keep active. Trying alternate types of activity, such as a pool program where exercises are done in water, can help lessen some of the patient's weight and allow him or her to move more freely. Walking in shopping malls can provide a venue for exercise even in cold and snowy areas of the country. No matter what type of exercise the patient prefers, finding the one that will keep the patient moving and exercising is the best option to keep the positive momentum going after a surgical procedure.

References

1. American Pain Society. *Principles of Analgesic Use in the Treatment of Acute Pain and Cancer Pain.* Glenview, Ill: The Society; 2008.

2. D'Arcy Y. *Pain Management: Evidence based Tools and Techniques for Nursing Professionals.* Marblehead, Mass: HcPro; 2007.

3. Ashburn M, Caplan R, Carr D, Connis R, Ginsberg B, Green C. Practice guidelines for acute pain management in the perioperative setting. *Anesthesiol.* 2004;100(6):1–15.

Chapter 11

Comorbidities in Pain Management

Bill McCarberg

The majority of patients with low back and neck pain have comorbid mood disorders. Physical and emotional stability can be lost as pain erodes the individual's ability to maintain a sense of identity. Conflict presents when lacking objective tissue pathology, we seek to explain the pain in terms of patients' psychopathology.

Rather than attempt to determine whether pain or mood is more important, both should be identified and treated. Medical illness does not exclude psychiatric illness. Medically ill patients are much more likely to have psychiatric illness than patients without medical illness. Similarly, psychiatric illness with associated health behaviors often accompanies medical illness. Primary mood disorders also have a high incidence of chronic pain.

Psychological interventions including medications for chronic pain are rarely effective in isolation from somatic treatments. Distress, disuse, and disability accompany chronic pain problems requiring clinical attention. Even with excellent care of the somatic complaints, neglect of the psychological components can result in treatment failure. Psychiatric diagnosis such as depression can be helpful to the clinician and the patient by pointing to specific effective therapies. Unfortunately, the structure of most clinical settings makes the integrated delivery of mental and physical health care difficult.

Comorbidity is defined as the presence of one or more disorders (or diseases) in addition to a primary disorder or disease. The prevalence of persistent pain and psychiatric comorbidities varies with the population being studied. Community surveys show that when a pain disorder is present, there is higher likelihood of comorbid mood disturbances (Fig. 11.1).[1] A professional athlete may only seek medical care for chronic neck pain when it interferes with performance. The prevalence of psychiatric comorbidities in the athlete is the same as the general population despite persistent pain. Long-standing pain after the repeated trauma of sports activities is understood and accepted. Likewise, a nursing home population may have high prevalence of neck and back pain yet may have little effect on mood. Expectations of aging and persistent pain influence the coexisting mood.

On the other hand, when patients present to primary care or are referred to pain management, the incidence of comorbidities increases. In a sample of 200 patients with low back pain entering a functional restoration program,

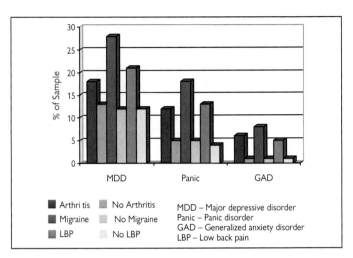

Figure 11.1 Pain and Mood in Community Survey. *Source:* From McWilliams LA, Goodwin RD, Cox BJ. Depression and anxiety associated with three pain conditions: results from a nationally representative sample. *Pain.* 2004;111(1–2):77–83. This figure has been reproduced with permission of the International Association for the Study of Pain (IASP). The table may not be reproduced for any other purpose without permission.

major depressive disorder occurred in over 40%. When there was more than one pain diagnosis, the prevalence psychiatric disorders increased to 59% (Fig. 11.2).[2] Depression in patients referred to pain centers varies between 55% and 87%.[3,4,5,6]

Mood disturbances can elicit pain; pain can elicit mood disturbances; either can exacerbate the other. Pain can make the mood treatment resistant; mood can make pain treatment resistant. There can be overlap in the presenting symptoms of persistent pain and mood as well. A Swedish study looking at 25 symptoms in 126 patients treated for peripheral neuropathy showed that many of the cardinal symptoms of depression are also seen as primary symptoms of pain (Fig. 11.3).[7] Normal motion during the night can disturb sleep independent of mood. Poor sleep can lead to lack of energy, poor concentration, and loss of interest in activities. Do these symptoms represent persistent pain or depression?

Patients with two or more pain complaints were much more likely to be depressed than those with single pain complaints.[8] The number of pain conditions reported was a better predictor of major depression than pain severity or pain persistence.[8] Addressing these issues is essential for optimal pain management since pain and mood diminish function and quality of life. The most common psychiatric comorbidities include depression, anxiety, and substance abuse.

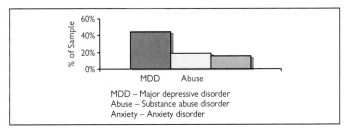

Figure 11.2 Psychiatric illness in chronic back pain. *Source:* Reprinted with permission from Polatin PB, et al. Psychiatric illness and chronic low-back pain: the mind and the spine-which goes first? *Spine.* 1993;18(1):66–71.

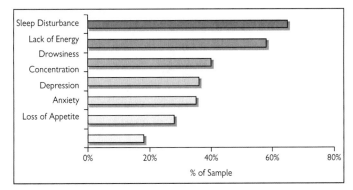

Figure 11.3 Comorbid symptoms in peripheral neuropathic pain. *Source:* Reprinted from Meyer-Rosberg K, Burckhardt CS, Huizar K, et al. A comparison of the SF-36 and Nottingham Health Profile in patients with chronic neuropathic pain. *Eur J Pain.* 2001;5(4):379–389, with permission from Elsevier.

Depression

Depression is one of the most common psychiatric comorbidities seen with persistent pain.[2] Patients often dismiss a depression diagnosis, claiming that the mood is a direct reaction to the pain. Physicians and patients often ascribe the loss of energy, decreased interest, disrupted sleep pattern, appetite disturbance, and social withdrawal to a normal reaction to severe pain and disability. The prolonged duration of these symptoms, however, may be indicative of a depressive syndrome. Patients may become defensive and not want to talk about feelings due to societal stigmas regarding mental illness and the portrayal of weakness.

Shifting the focus to psychological issues may threaten the patient, fearing that the examiner will conclude that the pain complaints are secondary to depression and not organic in nature. No clinical benefit is gained from the debate whether the depression caused the pain or the pain caused the depression. If patients meet the diagnostic criteria, it is likely that they can benefit from appropriate treatment.

Distinguishing between depressed mood and the clinical syndrome of major depression can be difficult. Depressed mood or dysphoria is not necessary for the diagnosis of major depression. It is common for patients with chronic pain to deny dysphoria but to acknowledge that enjoyment of all activities has ceased.

The diagnosis of major depressive disorder includes five or more of the following symptoms, have been present during the same 2-week period, and represents a change from previous functioning; at least one of the symptoms is either (1) depressed mood or (2) loss of interest or pleasure[9]:

- Depressed or sad mood
- Markedly diminished interest or pleasure
- Significant weight loss or gain
- Insomnia or hypersomnia
- Psychomotor agitation or retardation
- Fatigue, felling of worthlessness, or excessive or inappropriate guilt
- Diminished cognitive abilities
- Recurrent thoughts of death or suicidal ideation

It is important to recognize and treat pain and mood not only for the potential improvement in quality of life but also because chronic medical illness has been labeled a motivating factor in approximately 25% of all suicides. One survey shows that up to 50% of patients with chronic noncancer pain have contemplated suicide at some point.[10]

Pain is physically and psychologically wearing. Analgesics, antidepressants and anticonvulsants, and a sedentary lifestyle can contribute to fatigue. Pain and/or medication may impair concentration. Irritability, frustration, and dysphoria can parallel the level of pain.

Multiple tools are available to screen for depression, including the Beck Depression Inventory[11] and the Hamilton Depression Rating Scale,[12] and may be used at intake evaluation of pain patients.

Anxiety

Another comorbidity, nearly as common as depression, seen in persistent pain is anxiety disorders, including generalized anxiety and panic attacks. Anxiety has also been associated with somatic complaints, pain in particular.[13] It is closely related to avoidance of activities, which serves to promote ongoing pain, physical deconditioning, and social isolation.

Generalized anxiety disorder is defined as persistent and excessive worry or nervousness, present continually for at least 6 months and accompanied by three or more of the following[9]:

- Restlessness
- Fatigue

- Difficulty concentrating
- Irritability
- Muscle tension
- Sleep disturbance

The persistent pain may stimulate the underlying comorbid anxiety, making proper evaluation of the patient difficult. The same situation can occur as with depression where the patient fears the provider will conclude that the pain is secondary to anxiety, disregarding the primary pain complaint. It is unknown how much anxiety or panic contributes to pain or whether the anxiety is the result of the pain. It is also apparent that the anxiety must be addressed. Brief screening tools are also available for the intake evaluation of pain patients.[14]

Panic disorder is defined as a discrete period of intense fear or discomfort with at least four of the following occurring abruptly and peaking in 10 minutes.[9]

- Sweating
- Trembling or shaking
- Sensations of shortness of breath or smothering
- Feeling of choking
- Chest pain or discomfort
- Nausea or abdominal distress
- Feeling dizzy, unsteady, lightheaded, or faint
- Depersonalization
- Fear of losing control or going crazy
- Fear of dying
- Paresthesias
- Chills or hot flushes
- Persistent concern about having additional attacks
- Worry about the implication of the attack or its consequences
- A significant change in behavior related to attacks

Panic disorder is common and associated with high medical service use for unexplained symptoms since the patient believes this represents undiagnosed, life-threatening illness. Patients with panic disorder can receive extensive medical testing and treatment for their somatic symptoms before diagnosed and treated appropriately.

Substance Abuse

Many patients with chronic pain will be given abusable medications, including opioids, benzodiazepines, muscle relaxants, barbiturates, and amphetamine derivatives. The treatment is initiated to relieve suffering, yet behavior around the use of these substances becomes problematic. Early refills, escalating doses without approval by medical professionals, lost or stolen medication, and use with other nonprescribed substances (alcohol, marijuana) all present challenges for the clinician.

The diagnosis itself may be difficult based on *DSM-IV* criteria. Patients taking any of these medications may develop physical tolerance and physical dependence as defined elsewhere in this book. Tolerance and dependence have diagnostic implications in the use of illicit substances and alcohol. Tolerance and dependence also occur normally when opioids are used therapeutically to treat pain. The essential feature of substance abuse is a maladaptive pattern of substance use characterized by recurrent and significant adverse consequences. These include impaired role function, use in physically hazardous situations, and legal problems. It is distinguished from substance dependence in that it does not require tolerance, dependence, or a compulsive pattern of use.[9]

Treatment

Treatment of the psychiatric issues found in chronic pain patients starts with recognition of the comorbidities. Depression and anxiety can present with somatic symptoms including pain; pain can elicit mood disturbances. As stated earlier, pain can make the mood treatment resistant; mood can make pain treatment resistant. If not recognized, the comorbidity complicates treatment. Specific pharmacologic treatment for pain is discussed elsewhere in this text. Comorbid mood disorders may require referral depending on the expertise of the treating provider. Nonpharmacologic and pharmacologic options are available and patients often have the most benefit by combining more than one type of treatment.

Cognitive-behavioral therapy has been found to be effective in pain management and improving comorbid mood disorders. This type of therapy is usually done in groups involving multiple sessions presented by trained therapists. The focus of the groups varies with each session and usually follows the tenets listed next:

- Cognitive-behavioral therapy[15]
  - Modification of patients' thoughts, feelings, and beliefs
  - Commitment to behavior therapy procedures in promoting change (e.g., graded practice, homework, relaxation, problem solving, relapse prevention)
- Depressed and anxious patients focus on the following:
  - Somatic symptoms
  - Potential for ominous significance
  - Helplessness, hopelessness

Important principles to remember when considering pharmacologic options for comorbidities in pain patients is whether the medication will have a dual effect, treating pain and the comorbidity at the same time. There are multiple categories of drugs that are effective in chronic pain:

- Opioids
- Antidepressants

- Tricylics
- Dual reuptake inhibitors: serotonin and norepinephrine
- Anticonvulsants

These medications can be used effectively both in the treatment of pain and a variety of comorbidities.

Opioids

Opioids clearly have broad applicability in a variety of pain problems from neuropathic, nociceptive, acute, chronic, cancer, and noncancer pain. Opioids are among the most analgesic compounds known, yet they have other effects that motivate their use in pain patients. Opioids are anxiolytic in some patients and can quiet anxiety. In other patients opioids energize, relieving the psychomotor retardation of depression. Opioids also initiate sleep in many patients. Some chronic pain problems are typically worse at night (e.g., diabetic peripheral neuropathy); the sedation of opioid management may improve sleep.

Despite the improved anxiety, psychomotor retardation of depression, and sleep, opioids are not the preferred treatment for these comorbid problems. Nonpharmacologic measures are equally effective for sleep and do not impede stage IV and REM sleep as occur with opioids or benzodiazepines. Anxiety and depression management is better controlled with cognitive-behavioral strategies or antidepressant medication.

Buprenorphine is an opioid that is used to treat chronic pain especially when comorbid substance abuse is present. Buprenorphine tightly binds to the μ-receptor displacing any other opioid thereby antagonizing any attempt to add other opioids to the treatment, a benefit in an abusing population. Buprenorphine is also a partial μ-agonist with a ceiling effect. The result is analgesia for pain control. If the medication is increased beyond recommended doses, no increased benefit or euphoria occurs; another benefit in an abusing population. Chronic pain patients who improve in pain and function on opioids yet have trouble controlling their use of the medication may benefit with buprenorphine treatment.

Antidepressants

Multiple antidepressants have been shown to be effective for pain management when a neuropathic component is known or suspected. Most antidepressants with analgesic activity block reuptake of both serotonin and norepinephrine. The tricyclic antidepressants, especially amitriptyline, also increase dopamine and antagonize sodium channels. To what extent increased dopamine and sodium channel inhibition play a role in chronic pain is unknown. Serotonin norepinephrine reuptake inhibitors (venlafaxine, duloxetine, milnacipran) have shown analgesia in a variety of chronic pain patients and treat depression and anxiety. Highly selective serotonin reuptake inhibitors are effective antidepressants, treat anxiety, and panic disorder but have very little analgesic efficacy.

Given this profile of the antidepressant medications, it is expedient to use a medication to treat pain and the comorbid psychiatric disorder at the same time.

Anticonvulsants

Several anticonvulsants have shown to be effective analgesics in a variety of neuropathic conditions, including diabetic peripheral neuropathy, postherpetic neuralgia, HIV/AIDS neuropathy, and fibromyalgia. Gabapentin and pregabalin also treat generalized anxiety disorder and may improve insomnia. Due to the sedating effect, dosing of gabapentin and pregabalin is typically started at night. Pain and comorbid anxiety or insomnia can effectively be treated with a single drug rather than combining multiple drugs.

Despite the existence of guidelines for the workup and management of chronic pain conditions, including fibromyalgia,[16] chronic back pain,[17] and neuropathic pain,[18] treatment is always the most difficult aspect of care. Comorbid psychiatric conditions intensify pain and make treatment more difficult. Guiding principles in treatment include the following:

• Combining nonpharmacologic and pharmacologic options maximizes the benefits and minimizes drug toxicity.
• Use the lowest dose of medication that produces the desired analgesia and improved function.
• Initiate pharmacologic management based upon comorbid psychiatric conditions that may also be treated with the same class of drug.

Conclusion

Pain is a product of efferent as well as afferent activity in the nervous system, yet tissue damage and nociception are neither necessary nor sufficient to explain the presence of pain. The relationship between pain and nociception is highly complex. The traditional view that pain is caused by either tissue pathology or psychopathology is outmoded and too simplistic to explain known pathophysiology or observed clinical behavior. The medical system with primary care and specialty referral is a familiar and nonthreatening structure to pain patients. Psychological care for patients with chronic pain should occur within this medical treatment setting whenever possible. The medical system of care is the effective way to reassure patients that the somatic elements of their problems are not neglected. The evaluation and treatment of psychiatric comorbidities can add an essential and often neglected component to the conceptualization and treatment of chronic pain problems.

References

1 McWilliams LA, Goodwin RD, Cox BJ. Depression and anxiety associated with three pain conditions: results from a nationally representative sample. *Pain.* 2004;111(1–2):77–83.

2 Polatin PB, Kinney RK, Gatcherl RJ, Lillo E, Mayer TG. Psychiatric illness and chronic low-back pain. The mind and the spine—which goes first? *Spine.* 1993;18(1):66–71.

3 Kramlinger KG, Swanson DW, Maruta T. Are patients with chronic pain depressed? *Am J Psychiatry.* 1983;140(6):747–749.

4 Lindsay PG, Wyckoff M. The depression-pain syndrome and its response to antidepressants. *Psychosomatics.* 1981;22(7):571–577.

5 Krishnan KR, France RD, Pelton S, McCann UD, Davidson J, Urban BJ. Chronic pain and depression. I. Classification of depression in chronic low back pain patients. *Pain.* 1985;22(3):279–287.

6 Fishbain DA, Goldberg M, Meagher BR, Steele R, Rosomoff H. Male and female chronic pain patients categorized by DSM-III psychiatric diagnostic criteria. *Pain.* 1986;26(2):181–197.

7 Meyer-Rosberg K, Kvarnström A, Kinnman E, Gordh T, Nordfors LO, Kristofferson A. Peripheral neuropathic pain--a multidimensional burden for patients. *Eur J Pain.* 2001;5(4):379–389.

8 Dworkin SF, Von Korff M, LeResche L. Multiple pains and psychiatric disturbance. An epidemiologic investigation. *Arch Gen Psychiatry.* 1990;47:239–244.

9 American Psychiatric Association. *Diagnostic and Statistical Manual of Mental Disorders.* 4th ed. Washington, DC: American Psychiatric Association; 1994.

10 Fishbain DA. The association of chronic pain and suicide. *Semin Clini Neuropsychiatr.* 1999;4(3):221–227.

11 Beck AT, Ward CH, Mendelson M, Mock J, Erbaugh J. An inventory for measuring depression. *Arch Gen Psychiatry.* 1961;4:561–571.

12 Hamilton M. A rating scale for depression. *J Neurol Neurosurg Psychiatry.* 1960;23:56–62.

13 Simmonds MJ, Kumar S, Lechelt E. Psychosocial factors in disabling low back pain: cause or consequences. *Disabil Rehabil.* 1996;18(4):161–168.

14 Spitzer RL, Kroenke K, Williams JB, Lowe B. A brief measure of assessing generalized anxiety disorder. The GAD-7. *Arch Intern Med.* 2006;166:1092–1097.

15 Institute for Clinical Systems Improvement. Healthcare guideline: assessment and management of chronic pain. 3rd ed. July 2008. Available at: http://www.icsi.org/pain__chronic__assessment_and_management_of_14399/pain__chronic__assessment_and_management_of__guideline_.html. [accessed May 11, 2009].

16 Goldenberg DL, Burckhardt C, Crofford L. Management of fibromyalgia syndrome. *JAMA.* 2004;292:2388–2395.

17 Chou R, Qaseem A, Snow V, et al. Diagnosis and treatment of low back pain: a joint clinical practice guideline from the American College of Physicians and the American Pain Society. *Ann Intern Med.* 2007;147(7):478–491.

18 Argoff CE, Backonja MM, Belgrade MJ, et al. Consensus guidelines: treatment planning and options. Diabetic peripheral neuropathic pain. *Mayo Clin Proc.* 2006;81(4 Suppl):S12–25.

Chapter 12

Prescribing Opioid Medication Safely

Yvonne D'Arcy

Safe prescribing is a necessity for all prescribers. Recent statistics indicate that more than 3 billion prescriptions are written annually, and of these prescriptions about 1 billion require some type of clarification by a pharmacist.[1] The potential cost to the patient is also very serious. Using the same 2008 data the writer found that prescription errors seriously harm and in some cases cause death to 7000 people every year and cause injury to 1.5 million more patients.[1] When a prescription is being written for opioids, there are more considerations than just the basic elements of the prescription. The type of medication and the potential adverse effects coupled with the risk of addiction and dependency create an increased risk for the prescriber and patient.

As a response to the identified risk factors, the American Pain Society and the American Academy of Pain Medicine recently developed a clinical guideline to examine the evidentiary support for safe opioid prescribing and to make treatment recommendations. Using a panel of national experts from a variety of disciplines, the current literature was reviewed and practice recommendations formulated. These recommendations include the following:

Prior to starting chronic opioid therapy (COT), there should be a full history and physical, appropriate diagnostic testing, assessment of risk of substance abuse and misuse, or addiction.

Using a benefit to harm analysis, a trial of COT for moderate to severe pain, or if pain is affecting function of quality of life, is an appropriate approach if the benefits outweigh the risks.

Before COT is started, informed consent should be obtained, a COT management plan developed, and a discussion with the patient of treatment goals, expectations, potential risks, and alternatives should be conducted.

When conducting the trial of COT, the dose and titration should be individualized.

Methadone should be prescribed carefully, with initiation and titration being done by clinicians familiar with its use and risks.

Reassessment of patients on COT should be done at regular intervals and include periodic, random, urine screens, pain intensity rating, functionality, progress to therapeutic goals, adverse events, and compliance with the prescribed regimen. Urine screen should be obtained more frequently for patients who exhibit high risk or aberrant drug-related behaviors. For the purposes of the guidelines, aberrant behaviors are defined as "a behavior outside the boundaries of the agreed on treatment plan which is established as early as possible in the healthcare provider-patient relationship"[2]

For high-risk patients, such as those with aberrant behaviors, history of drug use, or psychiatric issues, COT should be used only if strong monitoring parameters are able to be maintained and help from addictionologists or mental health specialists is available.

When dose escalation, high-dose prescriptions, and aberrant behaviors occur, the prescribing clinician should perform a full assessment to address the cause. Consider opioid rotation if side effects are intolerable or inadequate pain relief results, and consider tapering or weaning opioid therapy in patients with repeated abuse or failure to progress with therapeutic goals.

The approach to COT should be multidisciplinary and include functional restoration, psychotherapeutic interventions, and other adjunct nonopioid therapies. Clinicians should counsel patient on COT to avoid driving when impaired and encourage minimal or no use of opioids in pregnant women unless potential benefits outweigh risks.

Safe Prescribing

Opioids are a viable option for treating chronic pain such as back and neck pain[3]; however, the recent back pain guidelines by the American Pain Society suggest limiting opioid use to those patients who have severe level pain or where quality of life is being significantly affected by pain.[2] In a recent survey of nurse practitioners ($n = 400$), survey respondents ranked fear of addiction as number two on barriers to prescribing opioids and increased fear of regulatory oversight was cited as third.[4]

In most cases when opioids are prescribed long term, the average patient taking the opioids does not become addicted. Over the years, however, it has become more apparent that there is a risk of addiction at some level in the general primary care patient population. Determining the extent of the risk is difficult with the current literature database. Some of the best data indicate that the risk of real addiction in mixed primary care populations of opioid naïve and opioid exposed patients is low, <5%.[5] Since there is very little research in this area, there is no definitive answer to the question of addiction in a general patient population.

The problem seems to be very real and there is an escalating awareness of the issue. As of 2002 it is estimated that 4 to 6 million American patients were receiving opioids.[6] Additionally, 12% of all medications prescribed in ambulatory care office visits were noted to be opioids. In contrast, admissions to substance abuse centers for narcotic (opioid) painkillers increased by 155% between 1992 and 2002, and the number of emergency room visits for narcotic (opioid) analgesic abuse increased 117% from 1994 to 2002.

A recent meta-analysis found that the incidence of addiction in primary care patients was 0.19% for a preselected group of patients who had never been exposed to opioids and 3.27% for a preselected group of patients who had a history of opioid abuse or addiction.[5] In another study of 800 primary care patients being treated for a variety of pain complaints, the incidence of addiction for the overall group was found to be similar to other studies where the addiction rate was between 4% to 6%.[7] This means that the vast majority of primary care patients are using their opioid medications correctly with a select few developing true addiction.

Prescribers who are providing opioids for patients need to adopt practices that can protect them from any enquiries into prescribing practices or regulatory review. Safe prescribing simply means that prescribing practices follow current national guideline recommendations and use standard techniques for screening and continuing opioid therapy for patients who require long-term opioid therapy.

Universal Precautions

Using a term from infection control, standardized guidelines have been developed to manage all patients with chronic pain, including low back and neck pain. These guidelines have been termed "universal precautions in pain management" borrowing the concept of "universal precautions" from the infectious disease model, suggesting that it not possible for clinicians to assess all risks associated with opioid therapy.[8] Therefore, it is appropriate to apply the minimum level of precaution to all patients utilizing this treatment. Steps from these guidelines include the following[8]:

- Make a diagnosis with appropriate differential diagnoses
- Psychological assessment including risk of addictive disorders
- Informed consent

Table 12.1 Opioid Prescribing

Opioid prescribing was positively influenced by:

- Having Medicaid or Medicare
- An office visit longer than 15 minutes
- Already receiving an NSAID

Note: NAMCS data from 1992–2001 indicates 59 opioids prescriptions per 1000 visits.

NSAID, nonsteroidal anti-inflammatory drug.

Source: Olsen Y, Daumit G, Ford D. Opioid prescribing by US primary care physicians from 1992 to 2001. *J Pain.* 2006;7(4):225–235.

Table 12.2 What Is a Safe Prescription?

- Includes a risk–benefit ratio analysis before a medication is prescribed for a patient
- Screening tools and diagnostics are used to help determine whether the medication is a safe choice for the patient
- Provides a clear readable prescription with clear directions for use
- The right drug in the right dose for the right patient

- Treatment agreement
- Pre- and postintervention assessment of pain level and function
- Appropriate trial of opioid therapy +/– adjunctive medication
- Reassessment of pain score and level of function
- Regularly assess the four A's of pain medicine
- Periodically review pain diagnosis and comorbid conditions, including addictive disorders
- Documentation

Using Screening Tools

Screening tools provide a good baseline for monitoring patient behaviors, detecting aberrant behaviors, and determining the risk of long-term opioid therapy. The following list demonstrates behaviors that are more or less predictive of addiction. Using tools to monitor the risk potential for using opioids will help the practitioner decide whether opioid therapy for an individual patient has a favorable risk–benefit ratio.

Selected Screening Tools

1. *Screener and Opioid Assessment for Patients with Pain (SOAPP-R)*—assesses for abuse potential using a 14-item self-report measure. A reliable and valid measure where a score of equal to or greater than 8 indicates a high risk of misuse or abuse.

2. *Opioid Risk Tool (ORT)*—screens for aberrant behaviors in patients using long-term opioids using a 5-item yes/no format self-report measure. Scores of 0–3 are considered low risk, 4–7 are considered moderate risk, and scores of 8 and over are considered high risk. Has excellent ability to discriminate low-risk form high-risk patients in both men and women.

3. *Diagnosis, Intractability, Risk, and Efficacy Score (DIRE)*—a clinician-rated scale with questions in four categories: diagnosis, intractability, risk, and efficacy. The categories are further divided into psychological, chemical health, reliability, and social support. A score of 14 and above indicates a patient is a good risk for opioid therapy and those with lower scores are not considered good risks for opioid therapy.

4. *Current Opioid Misuse Measure (COMM)*—a 17-item self-report measure to identify aberrant drug-related behaviors for patients on chronic opioid therapy. The COMM is a newer tool that can identify emotional/psychiatric issues, evidence of lying, appointment patterns, and medication misuse/noncompliance.[9,10]

Screening tools should be used as a part of the initial overall history and physical and diagnostic screening. Patients who score as a risk on these tools should not be excluded from using opioids, but they should be monitored and reassessed regularly and may need more frequent urine screening.

Table 12.3 Screener and Opioid Assessment for Patients with Pain (SOAPP-R)

		Never	Seldom	Sometimes	Often	Very Often
		0	1	2	3	4
1.	How often do you have mood swings?	O	O	O	O	O
2.	How often have you felt a need for higher doses of medication to treat your pain?	O	O	O	O	O
3.	How often have you felt impatient with your doctors?	O	O	O	O	O
4.	How often have you felt that things are just too overwhelming that you can't handle them?	O	O	O	O	O
5.	How often is there tension in the home?	O	O	O	O	O
6.	How often have you counted pain pills to see how many are remaining?	O	O	O	O	O
7.	How often have you been concerned that people will judge you for taking pain medication?	O	O	O	O	O
8.	How often do you feel bored?	O	O	O	O	O
9.	How often have you taken more pain medication than you were supposed to?	O	O	O	O	O
10.	How often have you worried about being left alone?	O	O	O	O	O
11.	How often have you felt a craving for medication?	O	O	O	O	O
12.	How often have others expressed concern over your use of medication?	O	O	O	O	O
13.	How often have any of your close friends had a problem with alcohol or drugs?	O	O	O	O	O
14.	How often have others told you that you had a bad temper?	O	O	O	O	O
15.	How often have you felt consumed by the need to get pain medication?	O	O	O	O	O
16.	How often have you run out of pain medication early?	O	O	O	O	O
17.	How often have others kept you from getting what you deserve?	O	O	O	O	O
18.	How often, in your lifetime, have you had legal problems or been arrested?	O	O	O	O	O
19.	How often have you attended an AA or NA meeting?	O	O	O	O	O
20.	How often have you been in an argument that was so out of control that someone got hurt?	O	O	O	O	O
21.	How often have you been sexually abused?	O	O	O	O	O
22.	How often have others suggested that you have a drug or alcohol problem?	O	O	O	O	O

(continued)

Table 12.3 (Continued)

	Never	Seldom	Sometimes	Often	Very Often
	0	1	2	3	4
23. How often have you had to borrow pain medications from your family or friends?	○	○	○	○	○
24. How often have you been treated for an alcohol or drug problem?	○	○	○	○	○

Notes: Assesses for abuse potential using a 24-item self-report measure. A reliable and valid measure where a score of equal to or greater than 18 indicates a high risk of misuse or abuse. Used as an initial screen.

Source: Reprinted from Butler SF, Fernandez K, Benoit C, Budman SH, Jamison RN. Validation of the revised Screener and Opioid Assessment for Patients with Pain (SOAPP-R). *J Pain.* 2008;9(4):360–372, with permission from Elsevier.

Table 12.4 Opioid Risk Tool (ORT)

The Opioid Rick Tool (ORT)

Item	Mark each box that	Item score if female	Item score if male
1. Family History of Substance Abuse			
Alcohol	[ ]	1	3
Illegal Drugs;	[ ]	1	3
Prescription Drugs	[ ]	4	4
2. Personal History of Substance Abuse			
Alcohol	[ ]	3	3
Illegal Drugs	[ ]	4	4
Prescription Drugs	[ ]	5	5
Age (mark box if 16–45)	[ ]	1	1
3. History of Preadolescent Sexual Abuse	[ ]	3	0
4. Psychological Disease			
Attentbn Deficit Disorder:			
Obsessive-Cornpulsive Disorder,			
Bipolar, Schizophrenia	[ ]	2	2
Depression	[ ]	1	1

Total ORT Score (sum of 1–5)
Interpretation of ORT Score
Low Risk (score of 0–3)
Moderate Risk (score of 4–7)
High Risk (score of 8 and above)

Notes: This screens for aberrant behaviors in patients using long-term opioids using a 5-item yes/no format self-report measure. Scores of 0–3 are considered low risk, 4–7 are considered moderate risk, and scores of 8 and over are considered high risk. Has excellent ability to discriminate low-risk form high-risk patients in both men and women. Used when aberrant behaviors are suspected.

Source: Reprinted with permission from Webster LR, Webster RM. Predicting aberrant behaviors in opioid-treated patients: preliminary validation of the opioid risk tool. *Pain Med* 2005;6(6):432–442.

Table 12.5 Diagnosis, Intractability, Risk and Efficacy Score (DIRE)

D.I.R.E. Score: Patient Selection for Chronic Opioid Analgesia

Score Factor	
Diagnosis	1 = Benign chronic condition with minimal objective findings or not definite medical diagnosis. (e.g. non-specific back pain). 2 = Slowly progressive condition concordant with moderate pain, or fixed condition with moderate objective findings. (e.g. back pain with moderate degenerative changes). 3 = Advanced condition concordant with severe pain with objective findings. (e.g. severe ischemic vascular disease).
Intractability	1 = Few therapies have been tried and the patient takes a passive role in his/her pain management process. 2 = Most customary treatments have been tried but the patient is not fully engaged in the pain management process. 3 = Patient fully engaged in a spectrum of appropriate treatments but with inadequate response.
Risk	(R = Total of P + C + R + S below)
Physiological:	1 = Serious personality dysfunction or mental illness interfering with care (e.g. severe personality disorder). 2 = Personality or mental health interferes moderately. Example: mild-moderate depression. 3 = Good communication with clinic. No significant personality dysfunction.
Chemical Health:	1 = Active or very recent use of illicit drugs, excessive alcohol, or prescription drug abuse. 2 = Chemical coper (uses medications to cope with stress) or history of CD in remission. 3 = No CD history. Not drug-focused or chemically reliant.
Reliability	1 = History of numerous problems: medication misuse, missed appointments, rarely follows through. 2 = Occasional difficulties with compliance, but generally reliable. 3 = Highly reliable patient with meds, appointments & treatment.
Social support	1 = Life in chaos. Little family support and few close relationships. Loss of most normal life roles. 2 = Reduction in some relationships and life roles. 3 = Supportive family/close relationships. Involved in work or school.
Efficacy score	1 = Poor function or minimal pain relief despite moderate to high doses. 2 = Moderate benefit with function improved in a number of ways (*or insufficient information – haven't tried opioid therapy or or at aduration too for legitimate trial*). 3 = Good improvement in pain and function and quality of life with stable doses over time.

For each factor, rate the patient's score from 1–3 based on the explanations in the right-hand column.

Total score — D + I + R + E

Score 7–13: Not a suitable candidate for long-term opioid analgesia

Score 14–21: Good candidate for long-term opioid analgesia

Notes: a clinician-rated scale with questions in four categories: diagnosis, intractability, risk, and efficacy. The categories are further divided into psychological, chemical health, reliability, and social support. A score of 14 and above indicates a patient is a good risk for opioid therapy and those with lower scores are not considered good risks for opioid therapy. Used for screening at the initiation of opioid therapy.

Table 12.6 Current Opioid Misuse Measure (COMM)

17-items of Current Opioid Misuse Measure (COMM)

1.	How often have you had trouble with thinking clearly or had memory problems?
2.	How often do people complain that you are not completing necessary tasks? (i.e., doing things that need to be done, such as going to class, work, or appointments)
3.	How often have you had to go to someone other than your prescribing physician to get sufficient pain relief from your medications? (i.e. another doctor, the emergency room)
4.	How often have you taken your medications differently from how they are prescribed?
5.	How often have you seriously thought about hurting yourself?
6.	How much of your time was spent thinking about opioid medications (having enough, taking them, dosing schedule, etc.)?
7.	How often have you been in an argument?
8	How often have you had trouble controlling your anger (e.g., road rage, screaming, etc)?
9.	How often have you needed to take pain medications belonging; to someone else?
10.	How often have you been worried about how you're handling your medications?
11.	How often have others been worried about how you're handling your medications?
12.	How often have you had to make an emergency phone call or show up at the clinic without an appointment?
13.	How often have you gotten angry with people?
14.	How often have you had to take more of your medication than prescribed?
15.	How often have you borrowed pain medication from someone else?
16.	How often have you used your pain medicine for symptoms other than for pain (e.g. to help you sleep, improve your mood, or relieve stress)?
17.	How often have you had to visit the emergency room?

Notes: A 17-item self-report measure to identify aberrant drug-related behaviors for patients on chronic opioid therapy. The COMM is a newer tool that can identify emotional/psychiatric issues, evidence of lying, appointment patterns, medication misuse/noncompliance.[18,19] Used as an ongoing screen.

Source: From Butler SF, Budman SH, Fernandez KC, et al. Development and validation of the Current Opioid Misuse Measure. *Pain.* 2007;130(1–2):144–156. This table has been reproduced with permission of the International Association for the Study of Pain (IASP). The table may not be reproduced for any other purpose without permission.

The Opioid Agreement

Opioid treatment agreements outline the conditions for a therapeutic trial of opioid analgesics. The expectations and obligations for the patient and the clinician are clearly identified and reviewed. Criteria for continued use of these medications and identification of aberrant behaviors are reviewed.

Elements of the opioid agreement vary in content, but generally they include the following:

1. Goals of treatment
2. Side effects of medications
3. Definitions of addiction, dependence, and tolerance
4. Rationale for changing or discontinuing medication
5. Expected patient behaviors

Examples of opioid treatment agreements can be found at http://www.npeweb.org. If the patient deviates from the opioid agreement, the clinician must decide on an appropriate course of action. There are several options that are currently being used:

- Discharging the patient from the practice
- Continuing to treat the patient without opioid analgesics
- Continuing to treat the patient with greater vigilance
- Referring the patient to a pain specialist or addictionologist

The treatment decision is based on a thorough assessment with documentation of treatment rationale and the current status of the agreement. If the patient is discharged from the practice, a discussion with the patient as to the circumstances that led to this decision must take place. Directions for opioid weaning, management of withdrawal side effects, and referral to an alternate provider, be that an addictions specialist or pain specialist, should be included in this discussion with accompanying documentation.[11]

Deciphering Urine Screening Results

An evaluation of patient risk and the current office policy determines the frequency of urine screening. A baseline urine screen with random screening is a common pattern. Patients who are at higher risk can be identified through the use of a screening tool such as the COMM, DIRE, or SOAPP-R. If a patient has demonstrated some aberrant behaviors or deviated from the opioid agreement, more frequent urine screens than the usual 3-month screen may be indicated.

Testing procedures can be variable, and a two-step urine screen is suggested:

- The first step is a general screen to classify compounds using enzyme immunoassay.
- The second step is a confirmatory process using a method of gas chromatography/mass spectrometry (GC/MS). This step can provide a higher specificity for compounds.

A positive urine drug test result is defined as the prescribed drug not present; presence of an unprescribed opioid, or the presence of an illicit substance. Cross-reactivity and false positive and negatives can confound the results of the urine screen and skew results. For example:

- Several quinolone antibiotics can potentially produce false-positive results for opioids by immunoassay, but they are not misidentified by GC/MS.

- Codeine and heroin metabolize to morphine, so both substances may be identified in urine following codeine or heroin use, resulting in a false positive for morphine.
- Hydrocodone can be metabolized to hydromorphone.
- Marijuana is not usually detected in the urine from passive smoke inhalation.
- Marijuana can be detected in urine after cessation of use for up to 80 days in heavy users.
- Cocaine may be present in urine for 2–3 days if used as a topical anesthetic in dental or other procedures, and medical records should confirm this.
- Coca leaf teas can produce false-positive results for cocaine.
- Poppy seed is the only substance that can cause a false-positive opioid result in GC/MS. (Poppy seed cake, bagels, muffins, rolls, and Danish pastry contain poppy seeds.)
- Vicks nasal inhaler, selegiline, and some diet pills can cause a false positive for amphetamines.
- Heroin is difficult detect due to a half-life of 5–30 minutes, resulting in false negatives.
- A small percentage of patients metabolize opioid, especially oxycodone, rapidly resulting in a false negative for this drug.[12]

When interpreting the results of urine drug screens, consider the possibility of errors and patient variability and repeat the screen if needed.

Documenting with the PADT

The PADT is a specialized chart note designed to aid clinicians in monitoring outcomes during long-term therapy for noncancer patients on opioid therapy. It takes only minutes to complete and should supplement existing documentation. The elements of the 4A's are the foundation of the tool and a final section requires the interpretation of the data to formulate an assessment of the risks (e.g., side effects) and benefits (pain relief, improved functioning) of continued therapy and designation of the analgesic plan (continued therapy, dose adjustment, discontinuation)).[13] Pilot testing of the PADT demonstrated that patients on chronic opioid therapy achieved relatively positive outcomes in terms of analgesia, functionality, and tolerable side effects).[14] Potential aberrant behaviors were common but viewed as an indicator of a problem in only 10% of the cases.

The elements of this two-page follow-up assessment tool include the following:

- Current analgesic regime
- Level of analgesia; average, worst, amount of pain relief from medications
- Activities of daily living; physical, family and social relationships, mood, and sleep
- Adverse events

- Potential drug-related behaviors
- Clinician assessment/impression of the opioid therapy
- Specific plan

The PADT is available through Janssen Pharmaceutical Products, LP, 2003. Elements of a safe prescription for opioids include the following:

- Date of issue
- Patient's name and address
- Practitioner's name, address, and DEA registration number
- Drug name, strength, dosage form
- Quantity prescribed
- Direction for use
- Number of refills
- Manual signature of prescriber

Understanding Aberrant Behaviors

Some patients who are taking opioids regularly to manage chronic pain can develop aberrant behaviors that may or may not indicate addiction. Some behaviors that are less predictive of addiction include the following: hoarding medications, taking someone else's medication, requesting a specific drug or dose, raising drug doses without a prescription several times, drinking more alcohol when in pain, smoking cigarettes to relieve pain, and using opioids to treat other symptoms. These behaviors may have a different source such as unrelieved pain related to undertreatment, or financial concerns. Some behaviors seem to be more serious and have higher consequences. Behaviors that are more predictive of addiction include concurrent use of illicit drugs, stealing or selling prescription drugs, injecting oral medications, repeated resistance to changes in therapy although there are clear negative effects, and deterioration in family and work relationships related to drug use.[15]

Further Reading

Butler SF, Budman SH, Fernandez K, Jamison R. Validation of a screener and opioid assessment measure for patients with chronic pain. *Pain.* 2004;112:65–75.

D'Arcy Y. *Pain Management: Tools and Techniques for Nursing Professionals.* Marblehead Mass: HcPro; 2007.

D'Arcy Y, McCarberg B. NP prescribing authority for opioids. *Pain Med News.* 2007;5(1):1,25–26.

McCarberg BH, Nicholson BD, Todd KH, et al. The impact of pain on quality of life and the unmet needs of pain management: results from pain sufferers and physicians participating in an Internet survey. *Am J Ther.* 2008;15(4):312–320.

References

1 Perrone M. FDA seeks plans from drugmakers to reduce misuse, harm from pain killing opioid drugs. *The Associated Press.* February 9, 2009.

2 Chou R, Huffman L. Medications for acute and chronic low back pain: a review of evidence for an American Pain Society/American College of Physicians Clinical Practice Guideline. *Ann Int Med.* 2007;147(7):505–514.

3 American Academy of Pain Medicine, American Pain Society. *The Use of Opioids for the Treatment of Chronic Pain.* Glenview, Ill: The Society (APS); 1997.

4 D'Arcy Y. Be in the know about pain management. *Nurse Pract..* 2009; |34(4):43–47.

5 Fishbain DA, Cole B, Lewis J, Rosamoff H, Rosamoff R. What percentage of chronic nonmalignant pain patients exposed chronic opioid analgesic therapy develop abuse/addiction and or aberrant drug-related behaviors? A structured evidence-based review. *Pain Med.* 2008;9(4):444–459.

6 Wilson-Fisher J. Strategies to stop abuse of prescribed opioid drugs. *Ann Intern Med.* 2007;146(12):897–900.

7 Flemming MF, Balousek SL, Klessig CL, Mundt MP, Brown DD. Substance abuse disorders in a primary care sample receiving daily opioid therapy. *J Pain.* 2007;8(7):573–582.

8 Gourlay DL, Heit HA, Almahrezi A. Universal precautions in pain medicine: a rational approach to treating chronic pain. *Pain Med.* 2005;6(2):107–112.

9 Butler SF, Budman SH, Fernandez KC, et al. Development and validation of the Current Opioid Misuse Measure. *Pain.* 2007;130:144–156.

10 Passik S, Kirsh KL, Casper D. Addiction-related assessment tools and pain management instruments for a screening, treatment planning, and monitoring compliance. *Pain Med.* 2008;9(S2):S145-S166.

11 D'Arcy Y, Bruckenthal P. *Safe Prescribing for Nurse Practitioners.* New York, NY: Oxford University Press; 2010.

12 Katz N, Fanciullo G. Role of urine toxicology testing in the management of chronic opioid therapy. *Clin J Pain.* 2002;18(4Suppl):S76–82.

13 Passik S, Kirsh K. Managing patients with aberrant drug-taking behaviors. *J Support Oncol..* 2005;3(1):83–86.

14 Passik S, Kirsh K, Whitcomb L, et al. A new tool to assess and document pain outcomes in chronic pain patients receiving opioid therapy. *Clin Ther.* 2004;26(4):552–561.

15 Fine P, Portenoy R. *A Clinical Guide to Opioid Analgesia.* New York, NY: Vendome Group Healthcare Division; 2007.

Chapter 13

Pain Management: Noninterventional Rehabilitation-Based Spectrum of Care

Steven Stanos

The primary care clinician serves a valuable role in assessing, managing, and facilitating a wide range of pain-related conditions. This role includes the assessment of acute injuries, for which appropriate assessment and treatment can be critical to patient quality of life (i.e., organ-related conditions, fracture, and musculoskeletal problems). A more disease-centered approach may be more applicable to chronic conditions where consideration of biological, psychological, and social issues may also be entertained. This chapter will review issues related to assessment and goals for acute, subacute, and chronic pain. A description of various allied health practitioners will be reviewed. Finally, tips regarding when and how to more effectively utilize referrals to other specialists will be discussed, including the role of pain management specialists, physiatrists, and addiction medicine.

Therapy Professionals

Proper referral to therapy professionals is an important function of the primary care provider, and like other clinical referrals made, can help to determine the success of an intervention and improved outcomes for the patient. Allied health professionals commonly used include physical and occupational therapist, pain psychologists, counselors, relaxation specialists, and nurse educators (Table 13.1).

Physical and occupational therapists are the principal members of the rehabilitation team that helps restore structure and function to injured patients suffering from painful conditions. Occupational therapy focuses on educating patients regarding proper posture and ergonomics related to functional activities. In some settings, occupational therapy may focus more on upper extremity disorders, activity of daily living, and work rehabilitation issues. Physical therapy may focus more on strengthening, stretching, and return to leisure and sport

Table 13.1 Pain Management Allied Health Team
Physical therapist
Occupational therapist
Pain psychologist
Relaxation therapist
Vocational rehabilitation specialist
Social worker
Recreational therapist
Others: music therapist, life coach, etc.

activities. Many times, therapists from different areas may work together or "co-treat" as a means of improving patient-specific outcomes with therapeutic collaboration.

Physical and occupational therapists employ the use of passive and active therapeutic exercises and passive modalities in guiding patients through the process of tissue recovery and rehabilitation. Targeted therapeutic exercises are utilized to address specific deficits in posture, flexibility, strength, balance, neuromuscular coordination, and endurance. Passive modalities such as cryotherapy, heat, and electrical stimulation are commonly used to address pain, alter tissue distensibility, and control inflammation. Patient and family/caregiver education may be an additional component of the long-term pain management program.

How Can Referral to Physical Therapy Be Successful?

Referring a patient with acute or chronic pain to physical therapy is common practice for all practitioners. A number of factors should be considered in order to better improve the chances of a successful outcome for the patient. Key considerations may include accessibility, timeliness for evaluation, level of skill and specialty training in the facility, appropriate delivery of services, and communication between referring clinician and the facility.

A referral to physical therapy usually includes an order or prescription for services. The referring document or order should include the patient's diagnosis, focus of therapy, duration and number of visits, and medical or physical precautions and/or restrictions. The initial visit usually consists of a comprehensive evaluation, which includes a condition-specific history and physical exam by the therapist. Prognosis and short-term and long-term goals are included in the evaluation report, which is usually forwarded back to the ordering clinician where the order can be signed off and /or modifications or suggestions can be made. In some states, a physical therapist may be licensed to practice without referral from a physician or medical practice. Therapy units are usually set on 15-minute intervals (units) where patients are seen individually for 1 hour (4 units). Progress, response to treatment, and monitoring of compliance are important parts of subsequent therapy notes that should be communicated back to the referring physician.

How Can I Make Sure Therapy Is Working?

Asking the patient to describe and demonstrate exercises or stretches learned in therapy can be an important part of subsequent follow-up visits with the clinician.

Example of PT Script:
Name:
Diagnosis:
Therapy:
Focus of Treatment:
Restrictions:
Number of visits, frequency:

A more appropriate facility includes therapists who focus on instructing and training patients in specific exercises, highlight the importance of patient compliance, and let the patient take a more active role in therapy. Facilities that rely heavily on excessive use of passive modalities (ice and heat packs, ultrasound, and massage) may not offer the patient any long-lasting benefits from a therapy program. Be cautious of facilities that include an evaluation by a physical therapist, but subsequent visits are done by a therapy extended provider (i.e., therapy aid), many of whom lack the experience to help coordinate and advance a patient through an active program. The therapist should assess and shape the treatment program to fit the interests of the patient but be mindful of psychosocial factors that may be limiting the patient's progress on treatment. The therapist should provide written instructions, exercise logs, and appropriate multimedia support to help advance the patients.

Pain psychology assessment and intervention focuses on both cognitive and behavioral factors related to pain. One's cognitions may impact mood, behavior, and function. Psychological intervention is focused on unlearning maladaptive responses and reactions to pain while fostering wellness, improving coping, perceived control, and decreased catastrophizing. Pain psychology interventions also focus on pain-related anxiety, depression, and anger.

Behavioral and cognitive-behavioral interventions include a wide spectrum of treatments focusing on changing behaviors, thoughts, and feelings related to chronic pain. These include traditional cognitive restructuring, behaviorally based activity planning and management, problem solving and skills training, relaxation training (i.e., deep breathing, progressive muscle relaxation), guided imagery, desensitization, and hypnosis (see Table 13.2).

Spectrum of Treatment Models

The primary care provider may utilize various allied health professionals to help improve acute and chronic pain patients' outcome. The primary care provider may be an important facilitator or point person for managing the patient-specific case or may use more structured multi- or interdisciplinary models depending on patient needs. Multidisciplinary and interdisciplinary treatment

Table 13.2 Common Components of Behavioral and Cognitive-Behavioral Treatment of Chronic Pain

1. Promotion of a self-management perspective
2. Relaxation skills training
3. Cognitive therapy: also know as cognitive restructuring or self-statement analysis, including behavioral experiments
4. Behavioral activation and management, including goal-setting and pacing strategies
5. Problem-solving skills training
6. Other interventions to change perception or emotional responses to pain, such as guided imagery, desensitization, hypnosis, or attention control exercises
7. Communication skills training or family interventions
8. Habit reversal
9. Maintenance and relapse prevention

Source: Reprinted with permission from McCracken LM, Turk DC. Behavioral and cognitive–behavioral treatment for chronic pain: outcome, predictors of outcome, and treatment process. *Spine.* 2002;27:2564–2573.

models are part of a continuum of medical care that ranges from a unimodal model of patient care to a completely integrative one. These models include, in order of increasing comprehensiveness and philosophical complexities: parallel, collaborative, coordinated, multidisciplinary, interdisciplinary, and finally, integrative approaches.[1] A parallel practice model involves multiple members working together with very defined and specific goals, many times not requiring direct communication to be successful. An example includes the various allied health and health care providers working in an emergency (i.e., phlebotomist, triage nurse, staff nurse, physician, radiology technician). Moving across the continuum, more collaborative models include a case manager helping to facilitate treatment between the patient and physician. More collaborative models involve less hierarchy and more communication between health care practitioners. Acute pain and musculoskeletal injuries may also be managed by a more simple collaborative approach. Chronic pain, however, necessitates a more comprehensive and collaborative model. In multidisciplinary treatment, the primary care provider may serve as the referral organizer, managing medication issues for a patient and referring to other professionals, such as physical therapy, for additional treatment. In multidisciplinary models, treatment is delivered at different facilities with minimal formal communication. This model is the most commonly used in the primary care setting, and relied on the primary care provider to manage most medication issues and make decisions regarding continuation of other therapies as well as possible referral to interventional specialists and surgeons. A more collaborative interdisciplinary model involves a number of specialists working in one facility, who are able to communicate and collaborate on an ongoing basis to better improve patient outcomes. This type of formal pain program is usually led by a pain physician or psychologist and delivered in an outpatient or inpatient setting.[2]

Overview of Mind-Body Techniques for Pain Management

Mind-body techniques are being more commonly used in the treatment of chronic pain conditions and include complementary and alternative measures (CAMs) and Western medicine–based approaches.[3] Common techniques in pain management include biofeedback, relaxation therapy, meditation, and guided imagery. A recent study of fibromyalgia patients found slow breathing reduced ratings of pain intensity, unpleasantness, and negative affect ratings in experimentally produced thermal pain.[4]

Biofeedback

"Biofeedback" refers to a mind-body therapy where instrumentation is used to provide "feedback" to the patient regarding a physiologic process. Biofeedback is a self-regulation technique that has been found to be effective in a number of chronic pain conditions, including headache and myofascial pain.[5] Biofeedback training techniques target pain-related bodily function such as muscle tension (electromyographic [EMG]), heart rate, blood pressure, and local skin temperature and conductance (i.e., sweating). These physiologic and measurable responses or "bio" are monitored and brought to awareness by the patient. Patients are given "feedback" of the physiologic response (i.e., breathing pattern, skin temperature, skin sweat, and muscle tension) by the trained therapist, and then learn to modulate those responses, many times as a means of creating a "relaxation response" or as a means of decreasing pain. As the patient learns the specific skill or technique, he or she continues to practice and improve the intervention individually.

Relaxation therapy uses similar "feedback" techniques to induce a relaxation response and include deep or diaphragmatic breathing, progressive muscle relaxation, guided imagery, and certain types of meditation and yoga. Some have divided these techniques into two categories, "deep" and "brief."

Relaxation Therapy

Deep relaxation methods include autogenic training, meditation, and progressive muscle relaxation. Autogenic training (AT) does not require tensing and releasing muscles but focuses on turning attention to muscle groups, suggesting feelings of "heaviness" or "warmth."[6] Attention is then focused on slowing heart rate and breathing. The overall goal of AT is autonomic regulation and muscle relaxation. AT may also incorporate imagery, for example, a patient imagining being in a peaceful place while imagining pleasant, not unpleasant body sensations, to help patients feel more comfortable. Another common deep method is progressive muscle relaxation (PMR), in which the patient focuses on tensing and releasing muscles, providing feedback to the patient and clinician of objective changes. As training progresses, patients develop an enhanced awareness of the body and a greater ability to relax more easily and in a shorter time frame. With mastering of the technique, fewer and fewer muscle groups are used and the patient can relax the entire body without "tensing."[7]

Brief methods (i.e., paced respiration and self-control relaxation) are utilized when the patient senses an acute increase in stress or anxiety. Techniques include self-control meditation (a shortened form of progressive muscle relaxation), paced respiration (the patient breathes slowly and deliberately for a specific time period), and deep breathing (the patient takes a deep breath, holds it for 3 to 5 seconds, then slowly releases it). The sequences may be repeated several times to achieve a more relaxed state. Deep breathing can be an effective tool in capturing and holding a patient's attention prior to initiating imagery and other techniques to distract the patient from pain, stress, or anxiety.

Relaxation therapies are easy to learn, utilize minimal health care resources, and are without side effects. However, they can be very powerful tools for the patient with persistent pain and elevated levels of anxiety and related muscle tension

Meditation

Some practitioners consider meditation to be a deep method of relaxation therapy. Although various forms of meditation are practiced, common forms include mindfulness meditation, transcendental meditation, yoga, and walking meditation. Mindfulness mediation is more commonly being used in pain medicine and involves the patient concentrating on body sensations, thoughts, or emotions that occur "in the moment." Some have described as a reframing of the experience of discomfort (i.e., pain or suffering) as the object of meditation.[8] The patient learns to observe these sensations and thoughts in a nonjudgmental way. Over time, meditation should be associated with less anticipation and negative view of pain. Yoga and walking meditation, derived from Zen Buddhism, focuses on controlled breathing with slow deliberate movements and postures. Transcendental meditation is similar but also focuses on a repetitive sound or thought, with the repetition of a word or sound.[9] As with relaxation therapies, meditation may be performed on a daily basis by patients with chronic pain to help maintain a basal level of pain control. It can also be useful in the management of acute or chronic pain "flare-ups."

Guided Imagery

Guided imagery begins with a relaxation exercise in order to focus attention and relieve tension. Common visualization of a safe place includes imagery of a peaceful location or more physiologically focused imagery such as imagery of fighting disease (i.e., white blood cells attacking cancer cells).[10] Verbal suggestions are then given to create a flow of thoughts that may focus the patient's attention on imagined visual, auditory, or olfactory sensations. A recent study found guided imagery with relaxation as a useful technique in a study of osteoarthritis patients, demonstrating reduced pain, improvement in mobility, and reduction in the use of over-the-counter medications.[11]

Referral to a Specialist for Additional Pain Management

Appropriate referral to a specialist is critical in patients with acute and chronic pain conditions. Early referral can include referral to a specialist for interventional therapies, acute surgical emergencies (i.e., acute organ pathology, herniated lumbar disc with neurologic deficits). Many times, after initial conservative measures have failed or offered minimal analgesic or functional improvements, referral to a pain specialist may be necessary. A number of additional reasons besides inadequate or suboptimal pain reduction may include comorbid psychiatric disorders limiting response to treatment, need for diagnostic evaluation, and /or validation of treatment plan. Referral may also be for consultative reasons (i.e., medication recommendations or nonpharmacologic recommendations). In management of acute and chronic pain with opioids, increased aberrant behaviors, problematic use of medications, or signs of addiction or medication misuse may be critical signals to refer the patient to an experienced medical management pain specialist for transfer of care or consultation. Early intervention and referral may help to limit the development or progression of chronic pain and related affective distress, as well as limited unnecessary suffering by the patient due to suboptimal care.

If initial interventions by the primary care provider provide limited or no benefit, referral to a pain specialist may be the next option.[12]

Table 13.3 Reasons for Referral to Pain Specialist

- Uncontrolled, severe pain
- Significant, ongoing disruption of physical and/or psychosocial functioning
- Comorbid psychiatric disorder
- Diagnostic evaluation for unknown etiology or complex pain syndromes
- Validation of a diagnosis and treatment plan
- Consultation for treatment recommendations
- Inability to establish mutually agreeable treatment goals
- Follow-up care to monitor opioid use/abuse

What is a successful referral?

- Significant improvement in pain relief?
- Improved clarity of diagnosis?
- Effective communication between patient and specialist?
- Details clarified or missed?
- Disability addressed?
- Function maintained or improved?
- Does the specialist communicate the plan of treatment and outcomes to you, the primary care provider?

Source: Haig AJ, Kesterson S. Chronic low back pain. In: Haig AJ, Colwell M, eds. *Back Pain (ACP Key Diseases).* Philadelphia, Pa: American College of Physicians; 2005.

Conclusion

The primary care clinician provides a valuable role in assessing, managing, and facilitating a wide range of pain-related conditions. A more disease-centered approach, common in other areas of primary care, that is, diabetes, hypertension, is needed for subacute and chronic pain conditions. The approach includes a more comprehensive assessment of pertinent biological, psychological, and social issues. A wide range of health care providers, including physical and occupational therapists, pain psychologists and counselors, vocational rehabilitation therapists, nurse educators, and other complimentary medical providers, may help the primary care provider develop a patient-specific treatment program facilitated by the use of theses team members. Pain psychology interventions may include behavioral and cognitive-behavioral approaches as well as mind-body-focused treatments. Examples of common psychological interventions include biofeedback training, meditation, guided imagery, and hypnosis. More specific to chronic pain management, professionals in the addiction medicine and behavioral health area may also be important areas of referral or collaboration. If the primary care provider feels ongoing referral or collaboration with other specialists is in order, referral to a pain specialist may be beneficial as a means of provider higher level care when transferring care entirely or temporarily to the specialist (i.e., for pharmacotherapy, multidisciplinary treatment, and to provide interventional therapies), or to better clarify the treatment diagnosis, medication use, and other questions the primary care provider may not feel comfortable individually assessing and treating.

Most important, helping to better teach patients to manage chronic pain condition relies on an emphasis that the patient assume a more active, rather than passive role, and all aspects of care, including the assessment, treatment, and subsequent adjustment in the patient's care. Many times, involvement of the patient's family, too, may help facilitate better outcomes and clarify any questions or concerns related to the patient's care. Again, focusing on biologic, psychological, and social issues throughout the patient's time in treatment will enable the primary care physician to provide more efficient, practical, and successful care.

References

1 Boon H, Verhoef M, O'Hara D, Findlay B. From parallel practice to integrative health care: a conceptual framework. *BMC Health Serv Res.* 2004;4:15.

2 Stanos, SP. Developing an interdisciplinary multidisciplinary chronic pain management program: nuts and bolts. In: Schatman M, Campbell A, eds. *Chronic Pain Management: Guideleines for Multidisciplinary Program Development.* New York, NY: Informa Healthcare; 2007:151–172.

3 Morone N, Greco C. Mind-body interventions for chronic pain in older adults: a structured review. *Pain Med.* 2007;359–375.

4 Zautra A, Fasman R, Davis M, Craig A. The effects of slow breathing on affective responses to pain stimuli: an experimental study. *Pain.* 2010;149:12–18.

5 Astin J, Shapiro S, Eisenberg D, et al. Mind-body medicine: state of the science implications for practice. *J Am Board Fam Pract.* 2003;16:131–147.

6 Luthe W. Autogenic training: method, research, and application in medicine *Am J Psychother.* 1963;17:174–195.

7 Jacobson E. *Progressive Relaxation. A Physiological and Clinical Investigation of Muscular States and Their Significance in Psychology and Medical Practice.* Chicago, Ill: University of Chicago Press; 1974.

8 Kabat-Zinn J. *Full Catastrophe Living.* New York, NY: Delacorte Press; 1990.

9 Astin J. Stress reduction through mindfulness meditation. Effects on psychological symptomatology, sense of control, and spiritual experiences. *Psychother Psychosom.* 1997;66:97–106.

10 Van Kuiken D. A meta-analysis of the effect of guided imagery practice on outcomes. *J Holistic Nurs.* 2004;2:164–179.

11 Baird C, Murawski M, Wu J. Efficacy of guided imagery with relaxation for osteoarthritis symptoms and medication intake. *Pain Manag Nurs.* 2010;11:56–65.

12 Haig AJ, Kesterson S. Chronic low back pain. In: Haig AJ, Colwell M, eds. *Back Pain. ACP Series.* Philadelphia, Pa: American College of Physicians; 2005:317.

Index

139